GRUB

OTHER BOOKS BY ANNA LAPPÉ

Hope's Edge: The Next Diet for a Small Planet
(with Frances Moore Lappé)

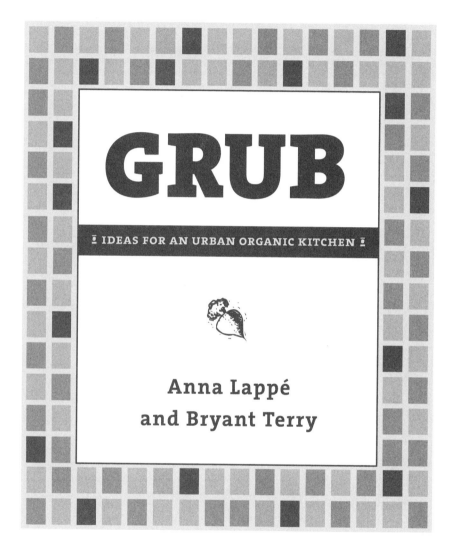

GRUB

⁛ IDEAS FOR AN URBAN ORGANIC KITCHEN ⁛

Anna Lappé
and Bryant Terry

JEREMY P. TARCHER/PENGUIN

a member of Penguin Group (USA) Inc.

New York

JEREMY P. TARCHER/PENGUIN
Published by the Penguin Group
Penguin Group (USA) Inc., 375 Hudson Street, New York, New York 10014, USA ·
Penguin Group (Canada), 90 Eglinton Avenue East, Suite 700, Toronto, Ontario M4P 2Y3, Canada
(a division of Pearson Penguin Canada Inc.) · Penguin Books Ltd, 80 Strand, London WC2R 0RL,
England · Penguin Ireland, 25 St Stephen's Green, Dublin 2, Ireland (a division of Penguin
Books Ltd) · Penguin Group (Australia), 250 Camberwell Road, Camberwell, Victoria 3124,
Australia (a division of Pearson Australia Group Pty Ltd) · Penguin Books India Pvt Ltd,
11 Community Centre, Panchsheel Park, New Delhi–110 017, India · Penguin Group (NZ),
Cnr Airborne and Rosedale Roads, Albany, Auckland 1310, New Zealand (a division of
Pearson New Zealand Ltd) · Penguin Books (South Africa) (Pty) Ltd,
24 Sturdee Avenue, Rosebank, Johannesburg 2196, South Africa

Penguin Books Ltd, Registered Offices:
80 Strand, London WC2R 0RL, England

Most Tarcher/Penguin books are available at special quantity discounts for bulk
purchase for sales promotions, premiums, fund-raising, and educational needs.
Special books or book excerpts also can be created to fit specific needs. For details,
write Penguin Group (USA) Inc. Special Markets, 375 Hudson Street,
New York, NY 10014.

Library of Congress Cataloging-in-Publication Data

Lappé, Anna, date.
Grub : ideas for an urban organic kitchen / Anna Lappé and Bryant Terry.
p.   cm.
Includes bibliographical references and index.
ISBN 1-58542-459-5
1. Natural foods.   2. Cookery (Natural foods)   3. Environmental protection.   I. Terry, Bryant.
II. Title.
TX369.L37   2005
641.3'02—dc22   2005054900

Printed in the United States of America
3   5   7   9   10   8   6   4   2

This book is printed on acid-free recycled paper ∞

BOOK DESIGN BY AMANDA DEWEY
GRAPHICS BY MATTHEW WILLSE
ILLUSTRATIONS BY TENJIN IKEDA

For my parents,
Beatrice and Booker Terry,
for nourishing me

BRYANT

For my dad,
Marc Alan Lappé
(1943–2005)

ANNA

Contents

Part Three

Menus

Resources

Figures

grub* (grəb), *n.*

1. Grub is organic and sustainably raised whole and locally grown foods;
2. Grub is produced with fairness from seed to table;
3. Grub is good for our bodies, our communities, and our environment.

*Grub should be universal . . . and it's delicious.

Foreword

Some people spend way too much time thinking about food. You know the type: a dozen kinds of olive oil in the kitchen cupboard, cranky when the goat cheese isn't served at room temperature, fond of restaurants that serve chocolate-covered edamame. When foodies and gourmands start talking about their latest culinary obsession, I look for the nearest exit. But most people don't spend enough time thinking about food, at least not in a meaningful way. They may worry about calories and carbs, and yet miss the real point. What we eat has changed more during the past thirty years than in the previous thirty thousand. Trans fats, genetically engineered soybeans, livestock pumped with growth hormones and fed slaughterhouse waste, Chicken McNuggets—nobody's ever eaten this stuff before. We've become a nation of guinea pigs, the subjects in a vast scientific experiment, waiting to see what happens when human beings eat too much industrialized food. Much of it tastes and smells pretty good. The pleasure, however, doesn't last long. Learning where our modern mcfood comes from and how it's made and what it's doing to the world leaves a bitter aftertaste.

Those are some of the reasons you should read this book. The authors don't want to lecture you or browbeat you into politically correct dining. They just want you to know what's wrong with our current food system and how easily it can be made right. They provide the basic information about how to eat in a way that's not only sustainable for the environment, but also for your body. The recipes here aren't too precious or fancy. I like the idea of food that's guilt-free and tastes good. The word *Grub* really says it all.

After this book appears, lobbyists for the fast-food and meatpacking industries will probably accuse Bryant Terry and Anna Lappé of being "food Nazis." That's one more reason to read their work. Bryant has spent years helping inner-city kids make the connection between a poor diet and poor health. Anna has been challenging the logic of industrialized agriculture since practically the day she was born. It makes perfect sense, in this age of doublespeak and disinformation, that they might be compared to Nazis. Meanwhile, the handful of corporations that control our food supply are wiping out small businesses, driving independent farmers and ranchers off the land, spending billions of dollars on deceptive mass marketing, pushing for everything everywhere to be the same, and attacking anyone who challenges their unusual version of the "free" market. The authors of this book may be passionate and committed, but if you're looking for the totalitarian impulse in America, just head for the nearest drive-through. The fast-food giants are becoming obsolete, and they know it. They're like angry, dying beasts lashing out. The twenty-first century doesn't belong to them. Now's the time for some grub.

ERIC SCHLOSSER

Opening Note

Bryant and I met because of a book. It was 2003 and mutual friends had just released the *Future 500,* a one-of-a-kind snapshot of 500 youth-led organizations around the country. Flipping through it, I stumbled on a description of the organization Bryant founded:

> b-healthy educates low-income youth . . . about healthy cooking, nutrition, and afford-
> able alternatives to low-quality food. b-healthy helps young people connect their personal
> health with the social and economic health of their communities.

I had only just moved to the neighborhood, but knew enough about the geography of Fort Greene, Brooklyn, to know that Bryant lived just a few blocks away. And I knew enough about him from this short description to know we had to meet. Within a week, we got together for coffee.

In that first meeting, we described the paths that brought us to food: His, from summers discovering the joys of food in his grandparents' backyard garden in Memphis when he was just "knee-high to a June bug" to a stint as a history Ph.D. student where he learned about the connections between poverty, malnutrition, and institutional racism. Mine, from a childhood in San Francisco as a test subject for my mother's *Diet for a Small Planet* to traversing the planet with her, researching social movements addressing the root causes of hunger and poverty for our book, *Hope's Edge.*

The idea for *Grub* emerged out of these conversations. We wanted to create a book that would explore the big ideas about food and farming and offer tangible steps and tantalizing recipes to create healthier lives for ourselves and the planet.

We wanted a book that would stir you to action—and stir up your appetite. For we may be living in an upside-down world—where food that is supposed to sustain us is making many of us sick, where farming has become one of the most wasteful industrial practices—but millions are trying to right it. And the good news is that righting it can be so simple, and taste so good. That's what this book is about.

Bryant crafted the seasonal menus and curated the cookbook section, bringing together food preparation tips, the poetry, and the musical inspirations. I developed and wrote Parts One through Three and distilled the resources at the back of the book.

We invite you to sit back and read—cook, eat, and enjoy.

Who knew what spark the *Future 500* would ignite; who knows what sparks *Grub* might.

Anna Lappé
Fort Greene, Brooklyn

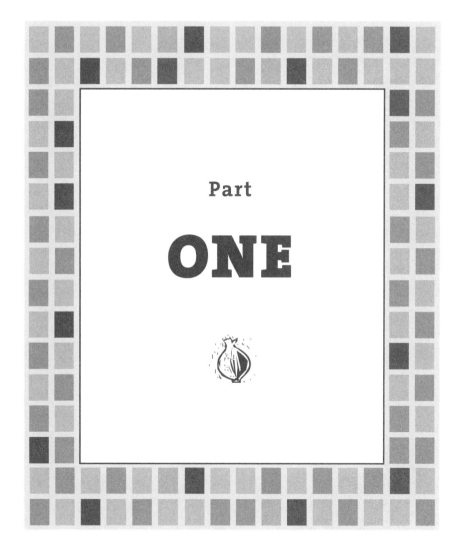

Part

ONE

ONE

The Six Illusions

When my grandmother was my age, her doctor suggested that to calm her nerves she might try smoking. She did. And she smoked cigarettes until she died. Now, nearly sixty years later, that doctor's recommendation seems like a failed attempt at dark humor, certainly not a prescription.

My grandmother's story is a small reminder that norms and knowledge can change, and do. They can change in one lifetime. In many ways, they already have.

Maybe someday—in fifty years, or thirty, or maybe even ten—we'll look back on what will have been be a relatively short-lived and ill-fated experiment: American-style industrial farming and our processed food diet. We will wonder, how could it ever have been so?

In the 1970s, power-suit-clad women stared out from the pages of glossies, dangling skinny cigarettes from well-manicured hands. Below, a tagline read: "You've come a long way, baby." We've come a long way, too, when it comes to what we're growing and eating. But maybe like the women in those ads, this particular progress is turning out not to be progress at all.

A few months ago, in the dead of winter, I found myself in Salt Lake City, surrounded by snow-peaked mountains and bracing cold. Friends I was staying with came home from a marathon trip to Costco with shopping bags overflowing. Plunking down a carton of chemically grown strawberries "fresh" from Chile on their counter, they somewhat defiantly asked me, What's wrong with this picture? Aren't our bursting-at-the-seams superstores evidence we're doing something right? Who would complain about strawberries in winter, or the abundance of our mega stores? But of course it's what we don't see that's worrying.

When novelist Barbara Kingsolver recently took up farming, some suggested it was an odd thing for a middle-aged woman to do. Her response?

> If a middle-aged woman studying agriculture seems strange, try this on for bizarre: Most of our populace and all our leaders are participating in a mass hallucinatory fantasy in which the megatons of waste we dump in our rivers and bays are not poisoning the water, the hydrocarbons we pump into the air are not changing the climate, overfishing is not depleting the oceans, fossil fuels will never run out, wars that kill masses of civilians are an appropriate way to keep our hands on what's left, we are not desperately overdrawn at the environmental bank and, really, the kids are all right.[1]

Kingsolver's words touch on the hidden devastation wrought, in part, by a set of choices we've made about growing food and feeding ourselves. The effects of these choices include:

- *Americans going hungry while food abounds.* More than 35 million Americans live in food-insecure households in which they are often unsure where their next meal is coming from.[2] That's as many people as the entire Canadian population. At the same time enough food is available to meet Americans' calorie needs almost two times over.[3]
- *Disappearing independent family farmers.* The United States has lost roughly a third of our farms since the early '70s.[4] And many of the surviving farmers are no longer independent, but are contract workers for large food companies. In addition, in seven farm states, over half the farms are no longer operated by farmer-owners, but by tenant-farmers who rent the land.[5]
- *Farmers' despair deepening.* Farmers are committing suicide at a rate double the national average.[6] Among farmers in the Midwest suicide is the fifth leading cause of death.[7]
- *Toxic pesticides blanketing the country.* Four pounds of pesticides for every American man, woman, and child are used every year in the United States, more than one-fifth of the world total for all pesticides and one-quarter of the world's herbi-

cides.[8] Yet crop loss to pests for some crops is double what it was before this chemical storm.[9]

- *Our diet making us sick.* The typical American diet is now implicated in diseases ranging from hypertension to certain types of cancer to Type 2 diabetes.
- *Our diet causing obesity and obesity-related disease to skyrocket.* With obesity rates soaring, as many as 365,000 Americans are now dying prematurely every year because of obesity-related illnesses.[10]

Few of us feel we're making these choices. We certainly don't feel directly responsible for most of them. Why not? In part, because we're blinded by this mass hallucinatory fantasy, one that is spun by six grand illusions convincing us that ours is the pinnacle of food and farming, that nothing is wrong with the status quo.

Living with these illusions, it's hard to see the solutions right in front of us. So the first step is to tease apart the pieces and see the illusions for what they are: ideas that have been intentionally spread for us to accept what we need not accept and acquiesce to what is actually in our own *worst* interest.

THE SIX ILLUSIONS

THE ILLUSION OF CHOICE	THE ILLUSION OF CHEAP
THE ILLUSION OF SAFE AND CLEAN	THE ILLUSION OF FAIRNESS
THE ILLUSION OF EFFICIENCY	THE ILLUSION OF PROGRESS

THE ILLUSION OF CHOICE

Peering from a taxi speeding along the always-under-construction Brooklyn-Queens Expressway, I spot a billboard two stories high. On it are pictured four bottles—Coke, Sprite, Dasani, and Fruitopia—and beneath them, one word: "Choice."

Choice. What's more American than that?

With the typical grocery store chock-full of more than 35,000 items, surely we've got it—

from those Chilean strawberries to kiwis from New Zealand to coffee from Vietnam. In just the breakfast cereal aisle alone, you can count a dizzying number of seemingly different choices. But do dozens of cereals or candy bars or sodas really equal *food* choice? To answer, let's back up and ask—what *is* food? Isn't it what nourishes us—what sustains life?

Well, yes, right? Then it is the choice for *real* food that we're losing.

Here's what I mean: Those 35,000 items in the typical grocery store are mostly manufactured products, manufactured with a single goal in mind: to bring the companies' shareholders the highest return. As I bring to light in the next chapter, once *that* logic kicks in, watch out!

The power of this profit motive has—in just a few generations—turned food into something else: processed products with sugar, fat, salt, and other additives pumped in and a lot of the essential good stuff taken out, and in which genetically modified organisms are nearly ubiquitous despite never having been thoroughly safety tested for humans or the environment.

This logic has turned food—essential to life—into something that is, literally, killing us, with estimates of up to 365,000 deaths and many more suffering every year from diet-related illnesses.[11] For many of us, we are among the first generations on the planet for whom the question isn't *whether* we will get the food we need, but whether *what* we eat will hurt us.

The sense of plenty we get from those mounds of winter strawberries or aisles of multi-colored cereal boxes can blind us to the real choice we're losing: diverse varieties of safe, locally grown fresh food. A hundred years ago we had 7,000 apple varieties; today, more than 85 percent of them have become extinct.[12] We've also lost more than 90 percent of the varieties of lettuce and corn.[13] Today, almost all of our milk comes from one breed of cows, most of our eggs from a single strain of hens.[14]

Genetically modified foods have narrowed our choices even further. Eighty-five percent of the soy grown in the United States is now genetically modified, as is 76 percent of the cotton, more than 75 percent of the canola, and 40 percent of the corn.[15] Though 94 percent of Americans agree that these foods should be labeled, as they are in most of the other countries that grow genetically modified foods (even China!), here at home we don't require labeling.[16] Can you have real choice when you don't even know what you're buying?

Without real choice, food has become anything but sustaining. Maybe now that, in this bizarre twist, much of our food has been made into a health threat, we need a new word, a word for what *is* nourishing for all—for farmer, for eater, and for the earth. To Bryant and me, the word is Grub.

Grub means real choice—and with it freedom—freedom from fear of food, from angst about weight gain, from worrying about who may have suffered to harvest our food. Grub means pleasure and health; it means food in tune with our cultural heritage. Grub is food grown without dangerous chemicals. It's fresh and seasonal, and processed under fair working conditions.

Grub is the choice most Americans are missing, and that more and more of us are wanting, and choosing.

THE ILLUSION OF SAFE AND CLEAN

When I learn that The Ritz-Carlton, Lake Las Vegas will be home to CropLife America's 2004 annual meeting, I assume the name is like one of those Chicago suburbs—Rolling Meadows, Crystal Lake, River Forest—places where there are no meadows, no crystal lakes, no rivers. After all, a lake . . . in Vegas? Vegas is desert country.

At the resort's turnoff, I see the golf course first: green grass dotted with palm trees. Sprinklers tick, spraying the thirsty lawn bordered by the original landscape: craggy rocks and dusty hillsides. Then I see the lake, or what turns out to be just a sliver of all 350 man-made acres of it.

At the hotel the landscaping is immaculate, not a leaf out of place, not a faux cobblestone unpolished. I can't help but notice, however, the uncanny quiet. There are no birds, no bees, no insects of any kind.

Clean. Tidy. Neat. That's what you see. What you don't see is what makes this artificial oasis in a desert possible: not only the water, but the chemicals, too. And you certainly don't see their consequences. Later, when I ask a property manager what chemicals are used on the area landscaping, she laughs and says, "Oh honey, I have *no* idea. But I'm sure there's a ton of it!"

The men gathered here (of the 269 registrants, only 17 are women) are leaders of the companies that manufacture virtually all our agricultural pesticides (BASF, Syngenta, Bayer CropScience, DuPont, and Monsanto, to name just a few) or representatives from the think tanks and public relations firms that promote them.[17]

Heading this chemical arsenal, these men are making decisions that affect the health— even the life span—of billions. No exaggeration.

True, humans have been experimenting with pesticides for centuries, but synthetic chemicals are a recent phenomenon. Many were born of war. When Swiss chemist Paul Müller discovered the insecticidal properties of DDT in 1939, suddenly the U.S. military had a quick fix for the devastating malaria and other insect-borne diseases that were wiping out military forces at home and abroad faster than enemy fire.[18] Within a year of its introduction into the civilian market in 1946, DDT was being used widely in U.S. agriculture.[19] Just five years later, sales of DDT had spiked tenfold, to $110 million.[20] Other wartime research led to the development of a range of toxic farm chemicals, including the herbicide code-named Agent Orange used in the Vietnam War to defoliate much of the country.

Crop dusting, which enables farmers to blanket large areas of cropland, was also, in a way, a child of war. After World War II, the government sold off more than 30,000 used war planes at a cut rate to farmers who converted them into crop dusters.[21]

Since World War II, the use and widespread application of synthetic pesticides (a term that includes fertilizers, insecticides, and fungicides) has soared. These man-made chemicals are now ubiquitous. Invisible to the naked eye, they're most likely used on your neighbor's lawn and your local playground. That golf course in the middle of the desert is probably blanketed with them, as is most of the cropland in this country, using a good chunk of the 1.2 billion pounds of active ingredients in pesticides sprayed in the United States every year.[22]

They're ubiquitous in our bodies, too. Centers for Disease Control research on our exposure to environmental chemicals has found that most of us are walking around with a significant "body burden" of chemical residues, including pesticides with known toxicity to humans.[23]

We're even born with them. In one study, an average of 200 chemicals and pollutants, including a number of pesticides—many known to be carcinogens or developmental toxins—were found in the blood of umbilical cords.[24]

There's now no place untouched; no child born chemical-free. Thanks, guys.

While standard setters have been battling it out over what constitute allowable levels of pesticide residues on food and how to determine the risk of extensive exposure to pesticides, at least a billion farmers, pesticide applicators, and farmworkers worldwide are our canaries in the coal mine—they are the ones who come into direct occupational contact with these chemicals. And we know they die more often than the general population of certain cancers, including non-Hodgkin's lymphoma and cancers of the skin, brain, and prostate.[25] They also suffer higher incidences of miscarriages and stillbirths, birth defects, and lower birth rates.[26]

For the rest of us, between 1 and 5 million people every year suffer acute pesticide poisonings, particularly children in low-income countries, with symptoms that range from headaches, fatigue, and nausea to paralysis and even death.[27]

Low-level exposure to pesticides—in the air we breathe, the water we drink, and the food we eat—has also been linked to a broad range of less acute, but often very serious illnesses, which may appear long after initial exposure. These include developmental disabilities and neurological disorders, such as Parkinson's disease.[28] These chemicals can also disrupt our hormones, weaken our immune systems, and decrease our fertility. Men living in rural Missouri, for instance, with detectable levels of metabolites from several common agricultural chemicals, have been found to have lower sperm counts than their city-bound peers.[29] Among children, for whom cancer is now the second leading cause of death, leukemia, non-Hodgkin's lymphoma, and brain cancer have all been associated with pesticide exposure.[30]

But wait. Don't we have government agencies to protect us—to make sure our food is safe and clean?

Yes . . . and, well, no.

When the bevy of agricultural chemicals flooded the market after World War II, the laws on the books—the 1938 Food, Drug, and Cosmetic Act establishing tolerances for pesticides in food and the 1947 Federal Insecticide, Fungicide, and Rodenticide Act requiring the United States Department of Agriculture (USDA) to register and properly label pesticides—were woefully inadequate to handle the demands for safeguarding our public health in a modern chemical era.

By 1969, 60,000 different pesticide products had been licensed by the USDA.[31] But "licensed" didn't necessarily mean safety-tested; testing was left up to the companies themselves. And at that time the agency had on staff a grand total of only one toxicologist, anyway.[32] Since then, pesticide use has continued to soar to 1.2 billion pounds of active ingredients annually, and much more if you count the so-called inert ingredients not officially tracked by the government.[33]

In film reels from the 1940s, you see nurses spraying DDT down the pants of children, kids sitting in dust clouds of the stuff, and soldiers as test subjects being sprayed point blank with it. At the time, we didn't fully comprehend insect resistance, or that chemical residues persist and travel, that they accumulate in the tissues of plants, animals, and humans and increase their toxicity, or that chemicals can be particularly damaging at vulnerable points in our lives (in the womb, when our immune systems are depressed, when we're elderly).[34] Now, however, we know all of this to be true.

We may not have known everything about the risks we were taking back then, but there were certainly early danger signs. By the 1950s, we started seeing insect resistance to pesticides like DDT, as well as epidemics of species that had been kept in check by their natural enemies before the introduction of insecticides.[35] As early as 1950, two Syracuse University zoologists found that DDT could disrupt hormones, observing that exposure to it "prevented young roosters from developing into normal males," and even speculated that "the pesticide was acting as a hormone."[36]

Then came Rachel Carson. Her book *Silent Spring,* in 1962, awoke a nation to the chemical revolution's impact on our health and the environment. Carson prophetically warned, "This pollution [from persistent organic pollutants] is for the most part irrecoverable; the chain of evil it initiates . . . is for the most part irreversible."[37] This "chain of evil" includes cancer, hormone disruption, and other illnesses. (In tragic irony, cancer took Carson's life just two years after *Silent Spring* was published.)

Sparked in part by the public outcry generated by *Silent Spring,* the Environmental Protection Agency (EPA) was founded in 1970. It took over the responsibility for registering new pesticides and evaluating and reregistering those already on the market.

Today, the EPA's position on the threat of pesticides seems unequivocal: "Laboratory studies show that pesticides can cause health problems such as birth defects, nerve damage, cancer, and other effects that might occur over a long period of time," according to its website.[38]

Clear words, yes, but the EPA rarely pulls a chemical from the market and even when it does, the chemical's toxic effect can linger. When the EPA banned DDT in December 1972, 675,000 tons of it had already been applied in the country.[39] With a half-life of fifteen years, DDT is still found in the environment, and in our bodies.

Instead of banning chemicals, the EPA generally pursues voluntary—and often feet-draggingly slow—cancellations or proposes "risk reduction" measures, such as user safety requirements, tamper-resistant packaging, and spray-drift labeling.

The case of benomyl is a chilling example. The chemical ingredient in a widely used DuPont fungicide registered for use in fifty countries on more than seventy crops, from rice, wine grapes, and mushrooms to nectarines, apples, and peaches, benomyl is suspected to cause cancer and has been found to cause birth defects in animal feeding studies.[40]

When benomyl was introduced in 1972, the EPA recommended that DuPont label the fungicide with a warning that it could cause birth defects; they didn't.[41] In the 1990s, the EPA proposed removing benomyl from the market because it was suspected to cause cancer; the company never did.[42] Instead, benomyl was okayed for use with EPA-determined acceptable residue levels.[43]

In 1990, a Florida woman exposed to benomyl while pregnant gave birth to a child with empty eye sockets.[44] (Benomyl had been shown to concentrate in the eyes of lab animals.[45]) Thirteen years later, her case against DuPont was settled for $7 million in damages, the judge ruling that the fungicide was responsible for the birth defects.[46] Still, benomyl was not banned. Instead, DuPont voluntarily pulled it from the market in April 2001, citing "business reasons" and complaining about the costs of defending "the product in the U.S. legal system where factors other than good science can influence outcomes."[47]

DuPont's decision came a full *twenty-nine* years after the EPA's first cautions about benomyl's health dangers. And even after DuPont canceled its production, existing stocks could still be sold for another year. At that rate, the EPA estimated that "all end use products should be used up in 2003."[48] So, correction: that would be a full *thirty-one* years after those first indications of threat.

Benomyl is not necessarily an isolated case. Though recent legislation has tightened standards for chemicals in farming, our guiding approach toward pesticide policies has seriously imperiled the EPA's effectiveness in protecting public health and the environment.

From the initial 1947 act, the governing guidelines in pesticide regulations state that pesticides can be sold or distributed in the United States if "when used in accordance with widespread and commonly recognized practice it will not generally cause unreasonable adverse effects on the environment."[49] Tricky language. It means that known hazardous chemicals can be registered as long as their instructions specify protections for the applicator and the guidelines specify acceptable tolerance levels. But putting instructions on a label doesn't mean they get followed, particularly by farmworkers who may be given no training or protective gear. And these acceptable levels of exposure don't account for what else happens in the real world (leaky equipment, accidental spraying) or in our real diet (multiple exposures to chemicals in the varied foods we eat). Plus, regardless of how it is applied or consumed, a chemical can still spread in the air, soil, and water.

How much is your life worth? To you and your loved ones, it is no doubt priceless. But when the pesticide law codified the health risks from pesticides (neurological disease, immune dysfunction, birth defects, reproductive failure, and more), it said such damages should be "balanced against economic benefits of pesticide use."[50]

A painstakingly slow reregistration process, this cost-benefit approach for approval and labeling—policies that permit toxic chemicals on the market—are just some of the drawbacks to our safeguards against pesticides. There's more. In establishing acceptable "tolerance levels" (basically how much of a pesticide residue is considered safe to remain on food or animal feed), we also disregarded, or misunderstood, fundamentals of toxicology. These principles of toxicology dictate that:

- **What's good for the goose may not be so good for the gosling.** The chemical industry likes to quote the sixteenth-century Swiss chemist Paracelsus: "All things are poisons. . . . It is only the dose which makes a thing a poison."[51] But Paracelsus didn't get it exactly right. Timing of exposure can make the poison, too. At certain times in our lives—when we're in our mother's womb, when we're infants and children, when we're nursing, or when we're elderly or our immune systems are depressed—even very low doses of certain chemicals, particularly endocrine disruptors, can wreak havoc. Setting uniform tolerance levels perilously ignores these big differences in susceptibility. It also ignores the differences in frequency and type of exposure—by air, through the skin or eyes.

- **Chemicals can mix it up, multiplying their toxic effects in our bodies.** By counting only dietary exposure and by looking at only one chemical at a time, pesticide risk assessment overlooks our overall "body burden"—the exposure to many chemicals from all of life's sources, from car exhaust to coal plants to our drinking water, which in combination can deliver a greater toxic punch.

- **"Inert" doesn't necessarily mean innocuous.** The EPA requires that only a pesticide's active ingredients (those responsible for the actual killing, repelling, etc.) be labeled and their usage monitored, though "inert" ingredients can make up as much as 95 percent or more of a pesticide.[52] What's the worry? "Inert" sounds like you, watching Monday night football, right? Not quite. While two-thirds of the nearly 3,000 inerts are classified as "unknown toxicity," many studies have already shown their potentially harmful effects on humans and wildlife. And more than 600 inerts are on the EPA's "List 4b"—considered potentially toxic if misused—and include everything from probable carcinogens and endocrine disrupters to dried mealworms and beer.[53] To make matters worse, we don't know which of these ingredients are where: hiding behind corporate "trade secrets," companies are required to identify (with a few exceptions) only the seven most toxic inerts. Says pesticide expert John Wargo, "A lot of toxins sneak in the back door with inert ingredients." (See the following figure for a breakdown of these lists.)

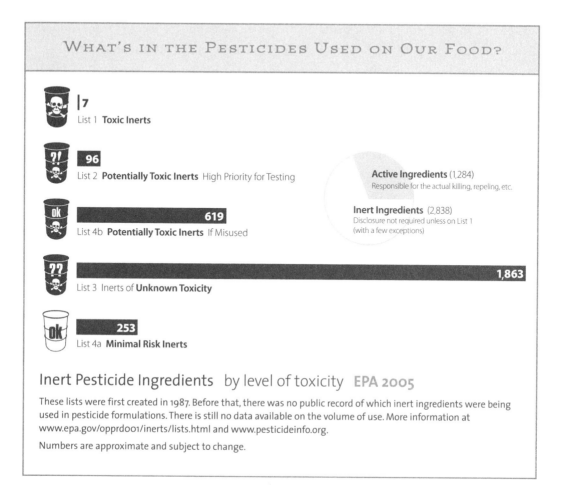

What's in the Pesticides Used on Our Food?

|7
List 1 **Toxic Inerts**

96
List 2 **Potentially Toxic Inerts** High Priority for Testing

Active Ingredients (1,284)
Responsible for the actual killing, repeling, etc.

619
List 4b **Potentially Toxic Inerts** If Misused

Inert Ingredients (2,838)
Disclosure not required unless on List 1
(with a few exceptions)

1,863
List 3 Inerts of **Unknown Toxicity**

253
List 4a **Minimal Risk Inerts**

Inert Pesticide Ingredients by level of toxicity **EPA 2005**

These lists were first created in 1987. Before that, there was no public record of which inert ingredients were being used in pesticide formulations. There is still no data available on the volume of use. More information at www.epa.gov/opprd001/inerts/lists.html and www.pesticideinfo.org.

Numbers are approximate and subject to change.

Recent legislation has begun to incorporate these complex truths of risk assessment. Landmark research in the early 1990s proved that children and infants are more vulnerable to pesticide residues because pound-for-pound of body weight children eat, drink, and breathe more.[54] Children also have more hand-to-mouth contact and more environmental exposure on playgrounds and in sandboxes, for instance. Their immune systems are also less developed and provide less protection than those of an adult. And they eat more of certain kinds of fruits and vegetables.

When the Food Quality Protection Act was approved in 1996, we finally had national legislation that considered the unique vulnerabilities of children and infants to agricultural chemicals and required, for the first time, additional protections for them. Also, the act considered not only the potential for pesticides to cause cancer but the dangers from endocrine disruption, too, with potential impact on fertility, intelligence, and the immune system.

But despite these enormous strides since our naïve love affair with the post–World War II chemical revolution, we still are bound by another important factor. Yes, there are rules and regulations, warnings and labels and websites with all kinds of information on them. But keep in mind what drives all of this: data. And the data the EPA uses to determine a chemical's safety comes from the manufacturers themselves. Yes, you heard me right: from the guys trying to sell you the products with the chemical in it. Sure, the EPA evaluates the data and has strict standards for testing, but if you compare manufacturers' findings with studies done by independent research, guess which studies raise fewer red flags?

Dr. Frederick vom Saal and Dr. Claude Hughes made just such a comparison of studies looking at the health risks of low-dose exposure to Bisphenol A, a common chemical used in everything from plastic baby bottles to pesticides to teeth sealants for cavity prevention. They divided studies completed in the past seven years into two categories: those supported by government grants or academic institutions and those funded by manufacturers. Among the manufacturers' studies (all eleven of them), none identified a problem with low-dose exposure to the chemical. And what did the independent studies—94 during the same period—turn up? Ninety-four percent found serious health effects associated with low-dose exposure, including spontaneous miscarriages and birth defects, hormone disruption, and certain cancers.[55] Yowzah! (Bisphenol A is an inert ingredient on List 3. Yup, that would put it in the "unknown toxicity" box.)[56]

Here's what we know for sure: pesticides pose risks, can make us sick, and in certain cases kill. In most aspects of life we don't take risks we don't have to, and we don't require definitive proof of exactly what a harm will be before evading it. Not so in pesticide policy: "We're proof of harm, not proof of safety, in this country," says Dr. Urvashi Rangan of Consumers Union. And the official word is we need more research to verify "proof of harm": as recently as 2000, the National Center for Environmental Health of the Centers for Disease Control and Prevention told a research team from the General Accounting Office that the "studies that have been conducted to date have been limited, inconsistent, and inconclusive"[57] and that "because of the complexity of the issues involved, it will be many years, and perhaps decades, before conclusive results from these studies are known."[58]

Precisely because we have scientific uncertainty—but the likelihood of harm—we need to incorporate precaution into policy. But taking an approach of precaution "turns our practice of science on its head," says Carolyn Raffensperger of the Science and Environmental Health Network and a leading advocate of the precautionary principle. Funny that the way we apply scientific knowledge has become so distorted that "turning it on its head" means applying common sense.

When in our lives are we willing to take *unnecessary* risk? It's risky to go darting into on-coming traffic, right? You wouldn't do it unless you had some really good reason—like to save your child. But we have no equivalent of a child darting into traffic when it comes to our food supply. At least with oncoming traffic, you can see the threat. The danger from these chemicals is invisible: you can't see the stuff, and you can still get hit.

There is no compelling reason to take the risks with chemical pesticides that we do. Consider, first, that many pesticides are applied just for "cosmetic" appearances—to make that orange with the flawless skin, the perfectly red apple.[59] (Let that sink in for a second. Maybe it's time we no longer equate smooth with clean.)

We also know there are less toxic alternatives to many chemicals—some made by the very same companies, but sold elsewhere. (Syngenta, the maker of atrazine, one of the most widely used herbicides in the United States, sells a less toxic alternative, terbuthylazine, in the European market, where atrazine has been banned.[60])

But more than just replacing toxic chemicals with their less toxic alternatives, we know that we can grow food effectively without the risk of the pesticides we use now. Well-documented analysis of organic farming flourishing in this country and elsewhere show the abundance of farms using ecologically sound approaches.[61] (These points are discussed at greater length in "Chapter Four: Grub 101.")

Worse, as you'll read, these chemicals have set us on a downward spiral of chemical dependence, actually further diminishing our long-term capacity to grow food.

At the CropLife trade association meeting in Vegas, I was allowed to attend only one session. It included a presentation by Stephen Johnson, then deputy administrator of the EPA. One of his first questioners asked how the agency was able to accomplish anything when it has "more than its fair share of fundamental extremists and aging hippies" whose mission is "to get rid of chemicals in the world."

That got a good chuckle out of the crowd.

Now I won't speak on behalf of EPA staff, but I think I can safely say that those questioning toxic pesticides are not "fundamental extremists," not trying to rid the world of every single chemical, but are simply promoting the radical idea that our food not only *look* clean, but actually *be* clean—and safe—inside and out.

THE ILLUSION OF EFFICIENCY

It's 1979. In a closed-door meeting of food executives captured by Frederick Wiseman's camera in the black-and-white graininess of his documentary *Meat,* one executive holds up a six-inch white plastic tube.

"Ten years of developmental stages at Cornell University. Four years ago we started to test-market it . . ."

"You mean the yolk is in there?" asks one exec.

Yup. "We take a dozen eggs and . . . take the yolk and put it in a very thin tube. We seal it and this goes over a continuous hot-water bath, which is cooking it. The centrifugal force . . . keeps the egg centered. When it comes out the other end it is completely cooked.

"We hold thirty-six patents. The equipment is very complicated. We put a dozen eggs back together again into one convenient form. . . . You can slice it and dice it and chop it. It eliminates all that cooking, peeling."[62]

Who knew executives had been searching for the perfect hard-boiled egg since 1979?

The persistent drive for greater efficiency—like getting rid of all that cracking, peeling, and slicing of hard-boiled eggs—has been the hallmark of this past century's industrialization of farming. And one particular definition of efficiency—getting more output with less input—has been a particularly powerful bludgeon used to trample sustainable farming. It's not efficient, critics say.

In 1962, responding to the publication of Rachel Carson's *Silent Spring,* then-Secretary of Agriculture Orville Freeman proclaimed that without agricultural chemicals: "Production of commercial quantities of many of our common vegetables would be drastically reduced. . . . Commercial production of apples would be impossible. . . . Commercial production of strawberries, peaches, and citrus would be impractical."[63]

Back then, industrial agriculture seemed to hold great promise. With new irrigation technology, pesticide promotion, and hybrid varieties of the Green Revolution, agricultural yields—output per acre—increased drastically starting in the 1950s.

Efficient, right? But let's take apart "efficiency." It's a concept that is only as meaningful as the factors you measure.

Industrial farming *looks* efficient (lots coming out!) because most of what goes "in" (or is used up) is not counted: fossil fuels, soil, water, pesticides, and, of course, labor. Nor is most of what *really* comes out counted: pollution, illness, destructive greenhouse gases.

Looked at this way, we can see that industrial agriculture is actually incredibly *inefficient:* reliant on fossil fuels in fertilizers, pesticides, and hydrocarbon-fueled irrigation, industrial farming uses up many times the energy needed in ecological farming. As more and more chemicals are needed to respond to increasing insect and plant resistance and loss of soil fertility, industrial farming has also trapped us in what Yale University's John Wargo calls an "addictive cycle of chemical dependence."[64]

Of this addiction, Stanford professor of biological sciences Paul R. Ehrlich wrote in 1978: "Pesticides are an ideal product: like heroin, they promise paradise and deliver addiction. And dope and pesticide peddlers both have only one cure for addiction: use more and more of the product at whatever cost in dollars and human suffering (and in the case of pesticides, environmental degradation)."[65]

We've certainly been victims of this addiction. Though we're blanketing the country with insecticides, we're having no easier time with the insects. While the volume of insecticide applied has increased tenfold since 1945, crop loss to insects has nearly doubled, up from 7 percent to 13 percent, according to the USDA's own data.[66] Introduced in 1945, insecticide use on corn, for instance, has increased one-thousandfold, yet over the same period crop loss from insects has increased, too, by 400 percent.[67] (And if you measure insecticides not by their volume, but by their toxicity, which has increased dramatically since the 1940s, you'd multiply use another tenfold or more.[68])

Organic farmers and their advocates have long argued that organic methods enhance resistance to disease and insect pests, while synthetic fertilizers and pesticides can actually increase crop susceptibility to pests. Decades ago, experts scoffed at the idea. "Now, twenty-five years later, research on plant systemic-acquired resistance is verifying virtually all of these observations," says Don Lotter, a leading expert on organic farming and agroecology.[69]

In interviews conducted for this book with organic farmers across the country, none said that crop loss to insects, pest management, soil fertility, or yields were among their biggest worries. And in a national survey of organic farmers, crop loss to weeds was seventh in a list of biggest concerns; pest and disease management was even lower.[70]

Even "problem" crops, such as apples and strawberries, that skeptics have long said could only be grown with chemical insecticides to protect their appearance are today successfully being grown organically. Farmers on a large-scale apple orchard I visited in Northern California had transitioned to organic and were no longer using a single chemical pesticide, relying instead on clever practices such as attaching to branches tiny twist-ties emitting sex pheromones, which confuse the male codling moths' mating patterns and prevent reproduction.

Strawberries are a notoriously fragile fruit, and strawberry growers use an arsenal of chemicals, including methyl bromide, a fumigant targeted by the 1991 Montreal Protocol for its ozone-depleting qualities and scheduled to be phased out in many industrial countries.[71] But in California I visited several organic strawberry farms getting by just fine without the stuff. The nonchemical solutions to key weeds and insect pests are both ingenious and basic. On an organic farm near Salinas, one nontoxic approach to weed management is simple: Black plastic mulch on the strawberry rows with holes poked through give the berries, but not the weeds, access to sunlight, eliminating the need for weed-killing fumigants and herbicides. Another innovation is field-length bursts of alfalfa planted every fifty rows or so, a nonchemical approach to deal with lygus bugs, which can destroy the skin of fresh-market berries. At the peak of the season, the bugs are drawn to the alfalfa, leaving the strawberries virtually untouched. For a farm this size, damage from this pest alone could run as much as tens of thousands of dollars a season. "With this trap cropping technique, crop loss has significantly diminished and the number of harvestable fresh organic berries in the summer months is way up," said Professor Sean L. Swezey, an entomologist at the University of California at Santa Cruz.

The wastefulness of our industrial food system is manifest not only in the overuse—and unnecessary use—of chemicals, but also in the production of factory-farmed meat. In *Diet for a Small Planet,* my mother, Frances Moore Lappé, details the process by which agribusiness transformed cattle, which had always been prized for turning nonedible stuff like grass into high-grade protein, into what she calls "protein factories in reverse."[72] Here's how it happened: By the 1960s, chemical fertilizers, hybrid seeds, and other new technologies had dramatically increased short-term yields. Without a correlating increase in people's capacity throughout the world to make effective market demand for more food, though, there was a glut of grain. The answer? Transform grain into a raw commodity for producing a more expensive item—grain-fed meat—and, voilà!, the invention of feedlot beef, one of the least efficient systems of food production that humans had ever created. To produce just one pound of steak requires sixteen pounds of grain and soy. On top of this inefficiency are the pesticides used, the antibiotics and hormones pumped into factory-farmed animals, and the water wasted. Raised on feed from heavily irrigated crops, feedlot cattle can use as much as 2,000 to 12,000 gallons of water for every pound of beef.[73] (Twelve thousand gallons is what an average American family home uses for all purposes in five months!)

If all this weren't evidence of our current system's inefficiency, consider what happens when food leaves the farm. A team of anthropologists and agricultural economists at the University of Arizona in Tucson spent more than eight years looking at what gets wasted from field to plate in this country. What they discovered startled even them: Of all food ready for harvest in the United States, 40 to 50 percent goes to waste every year.[74] In other words, nearly half of the food we could be eating never even makes it to our homes, let alone our bellies.

Efficiency loses meaning unless we consider all the costs and benefits. Sure, any business can turn a profit and appear efficient, if it doesn't pay its suppliers. Well, that's exactly what industrial ag does. And who are the suppliers? As we'll see in the next illusion: They are us taxpayers, and the earth.

THE ILLUSION OF CHEAP

Unless you shoplift your food—or dive for it in a Dumpster—you pay the amount on the price tag, right? Well, not exactly. See, what we spend at the checkout counter reflects just a sliver of the real cost of food. The price tells you only how much you must spend right there, right then, but it doesn't tell you anything about the "externalities" you also pay for. "Externality" is economics fancy-talk for the costs we as a society shoulder for individual and corporate actions.

So how much are we *really* paying for our food? One estimate puts the total cost of externalities related to industrial farming in the United States in the ballpark of $6 billion to $17 billion a year.[75] Their estimate includes calculations of the costs of:

- water pollution from agricultural chemical runoff and waste from factory farms;
- soil deterioration from pollution and loss of topsoil;

- impact of pesticides on ecosystems and human health (those counted are just the documented poisonings; many pesticide-related illnesses go unreported every year);
- pollution from the release of greenhouse gases from cropland and livestock operations.

Seventeen billion may seem like an impossibly high figure, but just think of one source of waste: Animals raised in U.S. factory farms produce nearly *one billion tons* of feces and urine every year—nearly four tons per man, woman, and child.[76] (California's Tulane County has the dubious claim of being the animal waste capital of the country: The county produces 21.2 tons of animal waste per person per year.[77]) That's a lot of you-know-what and it's our taxpayer dollars cleaning it up.

But even the $17 billion estimate undercounts every single one of the hidden costs of our food system. For we should also add to these costs the roughly $4 billion required to run the federal agencies in charge of regulating the food industry and mitigating these damages.[78] And we should add the costs we bear from misguided federal farm subsidies that add up to billions every year.[79]

We should also add the price we pay in oil. With their reliance on petrochemical-based fertilizers and pesticides, industrial farms in the United States use up 100 billion gallons of oil and oil equivalents each year in manufacturing our food—that's 338 gallons per person, per year.[80] And processing our food? Journalist Richard Manning calculates that we use ten calories of fossil fuel for every one we produce. A two-pound bag of breakfast cereal? It "burns the energy of a half-gallon of gasoline in its making," writes Manning.[81]

Another hidden cost is what our super-sized food has done to our waistline and our resources: Many of us are shelling out more and more of our hard-earned dough in diets and other fixes to alleviate our weight woes—from hundreds of dollars on prescription diet drugs to $3,999 liposuction procedures. Americans now spend more than $37 billion on dieting and diet-related products every year—that's 40 percent more than we as a nation spend on Homeland Security.[82]

The weight gain that gives rise to all this dieting has effects in surprising places. The ten extra pounds the average American gained in the 1990s requires the airline industry to use 350 million more gallons of fuel per year, costing the industry an additional $275 million annually.[83]

Diet-related illnesses increasingly burden our health-care system, too. Nearly one of every ten health dollars now goes to treat obesity-related medical problems, a significant toll on an already overtaxed health-care system.[84] And we each pay for this hidden cost for food as our health insurance premiums go through the roof.

The moral of the story? Even if you Dumpster-dive for your food, it doesn't mean it's free.

THE ILLUSION OF FAIRNESS

Growing up as Reagan babies, my generation was taught that fairness would flourish if we let the "magic of the market" work. Just get government out of the way, and competition will surge. We'll all be winners.

There's only one hitch. Ever played a game of Monopoly? Sure competition flourishes at first, but once someone corners the market on Park Place and Boardwalk, the game is as good as over. And we don't *all* win; some*one* inevitably does. Competition doesn't flower; it dies, and with it fairness itself.

In real life, as in the world of that childhood board game, competition and fairness depend on keeping market access open, on preventing a few owners from controlling so much that it's impossible for new players to get into the game.

In real life, this is not arcane economic theory. It's so obvious that long ago—the century before last—Americans put in place laws to protect us from the downsides of monopoly power and corporate collusion, starting with Senator John Sherman's Antitrust Act of 1890.[85] (Here, antitrust doesn't mean anti–good faith; it means anti–corporate conglomerate.)

Economists generally agree that once four companies control 40 percent or more of a market, real competition—what we consumers rely on for fair prices and practices—is shot.[86] With the 40 percent benchmark in mind, consider that:

- *In meat . . .* the four largest beef processors control 84 percent of the market, pork manufacturers control 64 percent, and poultry manufacturers 56 percent;[87]
- *In food processing . . .* the four largest companies process 63 percent of flour and 80 percent of soybeans;[88]
- *In commercial seeds . . .* four companies—Cargill, Monsanto, Novartis, and ADM—control 80 percent of the market;[89]
- *In GMO seeds . . .* roughly 90 percent of the market is controlled by one company, Monsanto;[90]

- *In pesticides . . .* six companies—BASF, Bayer, Dow, DuPont, Monsanto, and Syngenta—control between 75 and 80 percent of the world pesticides market. That's half the number of ten years ago;[91]
- *In retail food sales . . .* the top five supermarkets now control almost half of retail sales, almost double what their market share was five years ago.[92] Wal-Mart, which entered the food sales market only fifteen years ago, now collects roughly one out of three of our food dollars.[93]

This concentration of control over our food has huge consequences. It affects food quality as well as our bottom line; choice as well as fairness.

Senator Sherman must be spinning in his grave.

"In my neighborhood, I can buy designer gym shoes, every kind of fast food, junk food, all kinds of malt liquor, illegal drugs, and maybe even a semiautomatic weapon. But I cannot purchase an organic tomato," says LaDonna Redmond about Chicago's West Garfield neighborhood where she is a food justice activist, improving access to healthy food for her children and community.

In Paris, Missouri—where the population barely reaches 2,000—residents might have a tougher time finding a semiautomatic weapon, but an equal challenge finding healthy food. When I visited, I couldn't find a store selling fresh food of any kind, though the town is surrounded by prime farmland. My options? At Casey's General Store, a Midwest convenience store and gas station chain, I could defrost Tater Tots or personal-sized pizzas in the shop's microwave. At the local diner, I could order from a menu whose options ranged from hamburger to grilled cheese. Neither of my options is too local, or too healthy.

With the market concentrated into even fewer players' hands, people like Redmond and those in Paris, Missouri, have fewer real choices and low-income communities little recourse when stores decide to move out of their neighborhoods. In a study comparing regions in several states, researchers found three times as many grocery stores in wealthy areas as compared with poor ones.[94] In New York City, the wealthiest residents have five times as many square feet of grocery-store space apiece as do the city's poorest.[95] Adding insult to injury, grocery stores in low-income communities often jack up prices. In one San Francisco neighborhood, low-income residents paid 64 percent more for equivalent food than did residents in the city's wealthier neighborhoods.[96]

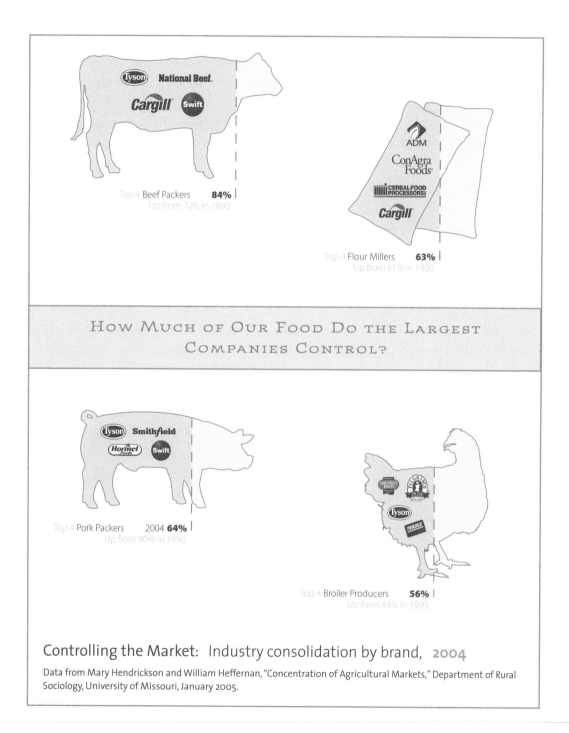

Top 4 Beef Packers **84%**
Up from 72% in 1990

Top 4 Flour Millers **63%**
Up from 61% in 1990

How Much of Our Food Do the Largest Companies Control?

Top 4 Pork Packers 2004 **64%**
Up from 40% in 1990

Top 4 Broiler Producers **56%**
Up from 44% in 1990

Controlling the Market: Industry consolidation by brand, 2004

Data from Mary Hendrickson and William Heffernan, "Concentration of Agricultural Markets," Department of Rural Sociology, University of Missouri, January 2005.

Then there's the impact of concentrated power on new businesses entering the market. Big food retailers now charge hefty slotting fees—fees companies must pay to get their products on supermarket shelves, which retailers say cover the costs of introducing new products.[97] A typical slotting fee can be up to $20,000 for one food item in one metropolitan area and as much as $2 million to introduce a product in stores across the country. In effect, slotting fees make it almost impossible for smaller companies' products to get into our shopping carts.

Consider the record (and I do mean record) of agribusiness giant Archer Daniels Midland, the world's largest grain processor. This company cheerfully represents itself as an upstanding corporate citizen, sponsoring public broadcasting and boasting in their latest motto, "Resourceful by Nature." Yet ADM agreed to a $400 million settlement for fixing market prices for corn sweeteners in 2004,[98] less than ten years after a top executive was found guilty of conspiring to fix prices for lysine (an additive in feed) as well as citric acid (a common food additive).[99] For that breach, ADM paid a $100 million fine, and three former ADM execs paid with prison time.[100]

All told, agribusiness accounts for 85 percent of recent fines imposed for global price-fixing.[101] Settlements like ADM's, however, are comparatively rare. Little wonder when government resources devoted to protecting us from monopolies—$211 million a year—is less than the typical budget for launching a couple new soft drinks.[102]

But price-fixing is not the only way ADM, and other food companies, unfairly pocket our hard-earned dollars.[103] When we buy Corn Flakes™, they get our money at the register—and then again on April 15th.

Here's what I mean: Every year, taxpayers underwrite the nation's farms to the tune of billions of dollars. In 2003, federal farm subsidies topped $16 billion.[104] Now, we often think of these subsidies as supporting Ma and Pa farmer somewhere out there in the heartland. The opposite is true. Nearly three-quarters of subsidies go to the top 10 percent of the biggest (and often most profitable) producers. In 2003, a few of these producers got more than $10 million each; one company received a whopping $68.9 million! While the average payout to the top 10 percent was $34,424 for that year, the bottom 80 percent received an average of just $768. Two-thirds of our nation's farmers got nothing at all.[105]

These subsidies actually *undercut* Ma and Pa farmer by helping the biggest producers grow food at below the cost of production and still make a profit. In the process, they pad the pockets of ADM and conglomerates like them. Thanks to these subsidies, ADM can buy corn and other commodities at artificially cheap prices, sell it for profit to food companies who in turn manufacture food products that are sold back to us for hefty earnings. Nearly half of ADM's annual profit comes from products subsidized by our taxpayer dollars or protected by the U.S. government.[106]

When some think of our nation's farmers, many still conjure up images of close-knit farm families, sustaining small-town America. But much of the independence of those family farms—and the fairness that there was in the farm economy—disappeared a long time ago. Now, many farmers no longer own their land; they rent it from corporations with headquarters in far-off cities.[107]

Even when farmers do own their own land, financial desperation is driving many to sign up as contractors supplying raw material to agribusiness. As contractors, farmers still technically own or rent their land, but they forfeit the freedom and self-direction real ownership brings. Virtually all poultry farms—and 85 percent of commercial vegetable ones—are now operated by contract workers for companies like poultry giants Tyson or Smithfield, which dictate every aspect of production, including variety, quantity, quality, delivery date, and price.[108]

While contracts pitch the promise of lifting the nerve-wracking risks of farming— unpredictable weather and prices—many farmers told me these contracts bring on whole new risks. Big debt is always perilous, and contract poultry farmers must take out loans of up to a million dollars to build the required facilities—*before* they even get their first contract. The company then determines the quantities of "inputs" (aka chicks) and how much they'll pay for the finished chickens. When contractors unexpectedly drop prices or refuse to buy a farmer's chickens, as they often do, there is no recourse. In most states, contracts require nonarbitration clauses: you sign away your right to sue.

Contract farmers must also agree to keep mum. "They can't talk to their neighbors about the terms of the contract; they're not supposed to talk to their bankers, their lawyers, even their wives," said Keith Mudd, forty-seven, a farmer in rural Missouri, and president of the Organization for Competitive Markets.

Forced into silence, farmers lose community solidarity and their capacity to work together for a fairer deal. They become, as one observer put it, effectively "serfs with a mortgage."[109]

"Most of the tools I have to farm I could do without," said Mudd, "but there's one indispensable thing I can't do without: that's a competitive marketplace."

In the first substantive Supreme Court decision to interpret the Sherman Antitrust Act in 1897, Justice Rufus W. Peckham ruled that "it is not for the real prosperity of any country that such changes should occur which result in transferring an independent business man . . . into a mere servant or agent of a corporation . . . having no voice in shaping the business policy . . . and bound to obey orders issued by others."[110]

Unfortunately, Justice Peckham, that's just where we're headed.

The Illusion of Progress

The lights were still dim in the University of Missouri meeting room, the PowerPoint was still humming, and the Ph.D. candidate's sweat had settled in above his glasses. He had just described a new experiment in genetically modifying trees to attempt to promote beneficial qualities for agroforestry. In conclusion, he said, "We wanted to know, could it be done?"

A friend sitting next to me whispered, "That's the problem! We're asking the wrong questions."

If looking back on several million years of human evolution teaches us anything about human nature, it is that we are constant innovators. As our tools have become more complex, so have our innovations. But we've evolved tools far faster than we have evolved an ethics of progress—a morality of technology. And we've developed technology faster than we have developed the safeguards to protect our common assets—air, water, soil, and more—from technology's unintended consequences.

We need not only ask, as the Ph.D. candidate so excitedly did, "Can it be done?" But also, as my friend went on to suggest, "Should it be done?" When some hear this caution, they assume it means stopping progress, but asking this question doesn't mean we *arrest* innovation, it means we choose the *best path* of innovation. It means we ask, "Is there a better alternative?" "What are the possible consequences?" "Who may benefit and who may suffer?"

After all, every choice is a matter of focus; every choice takes us on one path, away from another. Asking these questions helps take us on the path that moves us in the direction of the future we want.

Look at farming: The consequence of developing an agricultural system based on heavy water use, petroleum, and chemical pesticides—to fertilize the soil and fend off pests and weeds—has set off a cycle of wasteful production, petroleum dependency, and pollution, sickness, even death, unaccounted for when first introduced. The consequences of the decision to create our modern-day factory farms can now be smelled within miles from any one of them.

We've made these choices despite having the tools to grow food *without* these chemicals and inputs, to raise animals *without* the inhumanity and inefficiency of factory farms.

We would have even greater tools today if we had not placed a premium on a certain kind of agricultural innovation, that done in sterile labs with white-coated technicians. The result of this emphasis can be seen in the past century's farm chemical revolution and Green Revolution and its modern-day redux, genetically modified foods. And what a revolution it is!

First released in the mid-1990s, genetically modified organisms (GMOs) are now found in as much as 70 percent of processed foods in our supermarkets.[111] These genetically modified foods really refer to one specific kind of modification: their DNA has been intentionally altered with genes from another species. That means "crossing the species barrier and disturbing billions of years of evolution in the process," explains Claire Hope Cummings, a leading expert on GMOs.

"One of nature's fundamental constants has been the segregation and purity of the lineage of cells," wrote my father, Marc Lappé, a noted medical ethicist. In order to cross this barrier, food technologists must do some serious footwork, inserting a variety of other living organisms besides the gene they are crossing to introduce and activate the foreign DNA. These are some of the real troublemakers.

Genetically modified foods and these "add-on" organisms (including soil microbes and antibiotic resistance markers) worry many scientists and public health advocates for their potential to increase antibiotic resistance; affect the health of animals raised on GMO feed; foster weed resistance and super-pests; contaminate seed lines; damage wildlife and ecosystems and devastate biodiversity; deprive farmers of age-old control over their own seeds; and, perhaps most frightening, cause serious allergic reactions and illnesses, including some cancers, in humans. Some of these very concerns are already beginning to be documented.[112]

The crux of the problem with GMOs is the technology's fundamental misunderstanding of biology. The biotech industry, with its veneer of cutting-edge science, is actually founded on assumptions about genetics that are decades outdated.

Genetically altering organisms assumes that each gene corresponds with a specific trait, an assumption disproved by top researchers at the Human Genome Project upon announcing in 2001 that the relatively few human genes—30,000—could not possibly explain our organisms' complexity. After all, 30,000 genes are only about twice as many as found in a fruit fly, or a nematode worm.[113] Upon this discovery one project scientist said humanity should learn "a lesson in humility."[114]

The alteration of the genetic makeup of plants evidenced in GMOs is perhaps our greatest act of agricultural hubris. "What the public fears is not the experimental science," writes renowned cellular biologist and author Barry Commoner, "but the fundamentally irrational decision to let it out of the laboratory into the real world before we truly understand it."[115]

So why are we choosing this path, with all its risk and crude science? We need not dig much deeper than the financial incentives of the biotech industry to understand the motivation: They are, after all, seeking the kind of innovations that can be patented, trademarked, and sold.

In contrast, furthering sustainable, organic farming depends more on learning than buying. It means more research on interconnections—on plants and soil, insects and microorganisms— research that has been woefully underfunded by our government. Although the allocation is beginning to creep up, less than 1 percent of the USDA's budget for agriculture research has been going to explicitly organic projects each year.[116]

A look at the tactics of leading innovators in the field of biotech might give us additional pause. The companies developing GMO technologies, entrusted with the genetic heritage of our food, have been caught concealing potentially damning research, hiding serious mistakes, bribing government officials, even bullying farmers.

In May 2005, a 1,139-page unpublished confidential Monsanto report was obtained by Greenpeace under a European Union access-to-information law.[117] The report documented Monsanto research that found rats fed one variety of genetically modified corn developed statistically significant "abnormalities to internal organs and changes to their blood."[118] While Monsanto denied that these abnormalities were linked to consumption of the modified corn, public health advocates contend these findings raise further concern about the safety of these foods.

In March 2005, Syngenta revealed that for four years it had "mistakenly" sold hundreds of tons of genetically modified corn, not approved for human consumption, in the United States and abroad (the company wouldn't divulge to which countries).[119]

A few months earlier, in January 2005, Monsanto agreed to pay $1.5 million to settle charges and suspend prosecution on allegations of bribing Indonesian government officials a few years earlier to bypass environmental screenings of their genetically modified cotton before introducing the crop in the country.[120]

Monsanto has also been going after the farmers, spending $10 million a year and employing a staff of seventy-five to investigate and prosecute farmers for allegedly illegal use of their seeds.[121] As of May 2003, the company had filed lawsuits against 186 farmers, small businesses, or farm companies.[122] Many of these farmers deny they intentionally broke patent laws, claiming their fields were contaminated by drift or seed supply containing GMOs unbeknownst to them. Of those cases with recorded judgments, the average paid by farmers is close to $170,000.[123]

These examples point to a more sinister side of this so-called progress: Sure, we *can* invent a lot of things—that Ph.D. candidate may have had some really great ideas—but who is doing the inventing and toward what ends? Real progress is coming to a shared understanding of our values and seeking out paths, not of greatest profit for the few, but of greatest benefit to the many.

We're being sold the idea that our industrial approach to farming—with the latest genetically modified twist—is the avatar of progress, but sorry, folks, this might just be the grandest illusion of all.

TWO

The (Not So) Great American Experiment

THE EXPERIMENT

"Has he asked for anything special?" asks a doctor about Woody Allen's character, a health food store owner revived from two hundred years of cryostasis in the 1973 film *Sleeper*.

"Yes, this morning for breakfast he requested something called wheat germ, organic honey, and Tiger's Milk."

"Oh, yes, those are the charmed substances that some years ago were thought to contain life-preserving properties."

"You mean there was no deep [frying]? No steak or cream pies or hot fudge?" the doctor responds.

"Those were thought to be unhealthy, precisely the opposite of what we now know to be true."

"Incredible," concludes the first doctor.

Woody Allen—and apparently his audience—got the joke: wouldn't we all dream of waking up in a future where steak, cream pies, and hot fudge turn out to be good for us?

It was the 1970s and many people knew how wrong that was. The health food messages of the ecology movement were spreading; back-to-the-landers were "getting in touch with nature."

Chefs like Alice Waters of Chez Panisse were birthing what has become a celebrated organics cuisine and people like my mother were questioning the meat-and-potatoes American diet (and, in my mother's case, devising vegetarian concoctions in a book that would go on to reach millions).

But wait . . . what happened?

Fast-forward thirty years. While some of those health messages have moved from hippie fringe to mainstream normalcy, our national diet has moved in the opposite direction. Today the market for natural foods, which includes organics, may have what industry calls a 94 percent "household penetration" rate, but this doesn't say much about the dominant trend.[1] The big change since I was a kid? The degree to which we've become entrenched in the land of processed, super-sized fast food. There's been a dietary revolution, essentially within one generation; it's been a grand experiment and we are the test subjects.

One of my favorite chapters of my mother's *Diet for a Small Planet* is called "Who Asked for Froot Loops?" It's really quite a good question. Sure, as kids we may have asked for them, but we certainly didn't ask for them to be *invented.* Froot Loops, like most packaged cereal, is chock-full of high-fructose corn syrup, additives, and more. The cereal's tempting sweetness, image, and branding—even I was a sucker for Toucan Sam—allow the company to get away with charging mega bucks for what are, really, some of the cheapest ingredients around (cheap in part because we taxpayers subsidize them).

It's as if someone asked, What would happen if we decided what food to grow and feed the country based not on the greatest health return to all of us, but on highest financial return to a few?

Well, we've found out. Within a blink of the historic eye, we've turned away from the diet our bodies evolved on, a diet rich in whole grains and fruits and vegetables, with animal fat and protein playing a complementary role. Our prehistoric ancestors may have eaten some meat (and certainly insects), Jane Goodall and Gary McAvoy tell us in *Harvest of Hope,* but plants were likely to have made up most of their overall diet.[2] And our nearest ancestral relatives? Goodall found that among the chimpanzees she studied in Gombe, Tanzania, meat made up only 2 percent of their diet.

So we've replaced this diet we evolved eating with one heavy on factory-farmed meat and full of high-fat, high-sugar, high-salt, and highly processed foods—in effect turning nutritional wisdom on its head. This dietary experiment is playing itself out in the bodies of millions of us every day, and the guinea pigs are not faring too well.

THE ANTI-GRUB DIET

Imagine New York City in the year 2022: The population has hit 40 million plus. The sweltering heat from full-scale global warming nearly melts the skin, and one corporation, Soylent, controls half the world's food supply. A jar of strawberry jam will run you $150 and the starving masses survive on chips of Soylent Yellow, Red, and—the latest—Green. That's at least how Charlton Heston's 1973 flick *Soylent Green* pictured it.

The kicker (and don't read this if you want to keep the suspense) is what Soylent Green is. Heston gets dragged off-screen at the film's end shouting his horrific discovery to anyone who will listen: "Soylent Green—it's people!"

Okay, so eating concentrated cubes of people is still a wildly extreme vision of the future of food. But we have certainly witnessed a dramatic transformation of our diet from the whole foods we evolved on to highly processed victuals—from Pop-Tarts to Twinkies to Pringles. In many places, it is easier to find a Vitamin Shoppe with air-packed nutrients in powder form, or a fast-food joint with decidedly un-chicken-shaped nuggets, than it is to find fresh whole food.

Along with eating more processed food, we're also simply eating out more, much more. Almost half of our food dollar now goes to food consumed outside the house in fast-food, take-out, or sit-down restaurants.[3] Whether it's processed and packaged, or bought at one of these restaurants, food we don't prepare is more likely to be high-fat, high-salt, and high-sugar: added flavor on the cheap.

And we're just plain eating more, on average 300 calories more per day than we did in 1985. Almost half of these additional calories come from more refined grains, a quarter from more added fats, and another quarter from added sugars.[4] We're also consuming the all-new-to-our-bodies high-fructose corn syrup, trans fats, and factory-farmed meat that you'll read about soon.

These are just some of the defining elements of the anti-Grub diet. You'll probably recognize them, maybe even have eaten them. And if you look carefully, you'll see that each of these elements has padded a company's bottom line, while doing little for our health.

▼ LESS

Fruits and Vegetables

- Half of Americans consume less than one serving of fruit a day,[5] only one in five eat five servings a day.[6]
- The only vegetables on the rise are romaine and bagged lettuce.[7]
- In a nationwide study of infants and toddlers, half didn't eat a single vegetable for lunch, one-third had none for dinner. Fruit was missing from half of the breakfasts and lunches, and 60 percent of dinners. [8]

Variety

- Only three vegetables—iceberg lettuce, potatoes (frozen, fresh, and potato chips), and canned tomatoes—constituted nearly half of all vegetable servings in 2000.[9]

▲ MORE

High-Fructose Corn Syrup

- Consumption of high-fructose corn syrup has increased 4,000 percent since its introduction in the 1970s; the average American now consumes nearly 63 pounds of it annually, 15 to 20 percent of their total daily caloric intake.[10]

Factory-Farmed Meat

- We're now eating 223 pounds of meat per person per year, up from 177 pounds in 1970. All but a tiny percent of it is now raised in factory farms, fed on a diet that includes antibiotics and growth hormones.[11]

Oils and Fats (and Trans Fats)

- We're eating 38 percent more fats and oils than in 1970—600 calories' worth a day—and many of these are "bad" fats, such as trans fats.[12]

Sodium

- The average American now consumes twice the recommended daily amount of sodium.[13]

For Whom the Meat Tolls: Antibiotics, Hormones, and Pesticides

We may have the impression that as a nation we've moved away from the meat-and-potatoes American diet, but we're still eating a lot of potatoes (think French fries and potato chips) and a lot of meat, too: 223 pounds of it per person per year, nearly twice what we consumed in the 1930s.[14]

Yes, we've replaced some red meat with poultry and pork over the past few decades, but whatever type of meat it is, nearly all of it is factory farmed with animals raised in cramped confinement on diets of chemically grown grain, genetically modified soy, even animal by-products, such as fat, blood, bone, and fish meal.[15]

Most factory-farmed animals are also raised, nearly from day one, on growth hormones and antibiotics, even though scientists have raised concerns about both. Europe went so far as to ban the importation of hormone-raised American beef in 1985. In the late 1990s, a committee of European scientists reinforced concerns that eating meat raised on hormones may contribute to certain cancers and hormonal disruption in humans.[16] Under the European Union, the ban continues.

For decades, scientists here and abroad have also warned that overuse of antibiotics in factory farms is leading us toward a precarious future in which our best (and sometimes only) defense against certain bacteria will be dramatically reduced, if not rendered useless, by antibiotic resistance. As far back as 1982, my father, Marc Lappé, wrote a book about it, called *Germs That Won't Die: Medical Consequences of the Misuse of Antibiotics.*

Today, 70 percent of bacteria linked to infections in hospitals are resistant to at least one of the drugs needed to treat them.[19] Studies have found that people can be exposed to antibiotic-resistant bacteria in surface and groundwater contaminated with waste from hog factory farms and in retail pork products, and that people living near these factory farms can even be exposed through the air they breathe.[20]

Yet antibiotic use on factory farms continues to increase, with nearly three-quarters of all antibiotics and related drugs produced in this country going not to humans but to healthy animals.[17] That's right, *healthy* animals. See, most antibiotics are not used selectively for sick animals, but rather on a broad scale, across whole populations, to promote growth and to compensate for the stress of the overcrowded and unsanitary conditions of factory farms.[18]

Children of the Corn:
High-Fructose Corn Syrup

In 1970, high-fructose corn syrup hadn't yet been invented. More than thirty years later, chances are that just today you've eaten something that contains it. It makes up nearly half of the sweeteners used in processed foods and is found in everything from sodas and fruit juice to crackers and cereal.[21]

Developed in the early '70s by Japanese food scientists, high-fructose corn syrup instantly became a hit among food industry CEOs because it reduces their companies' costs. Why? For starters, it can be six times as sweet as cane sugar and is cheaper to produce in part because it's made from corn, which is heavily subsidized by our taxes.[22] When U.S. companies began using high-fructose corn syrup, profit margins of mostly sugar food items shot through the roof. Using high-fructose corn syrup saved Coke and Pepsi 20 percent in sweetener costs, boosting profits even as these companies boosted portion size.[23]

Industry has staunchly maintained that high-fructose corn syrup is processed by our bodies no differently from any other sweetener. The Food and Drug Administration concurred in 1983, granting high-fructose corn syrup the status of "generally recognized as safe" for use in foods and beverages.[24]

But it turns out our body *does* process high-fructose corn syrup differently from other sugars. Fructose is processed in our liver, and once there it triggers the liver's release of fat cells, or triglycerides. High triglycerides put us at higher risk for heart disease and stroke, and for putting on—and keeping on—the weight.[25] Scientists have also shown that the sweetener doesn't send the same "I'm full" signal to the brain as when we consume sugar.[26]

In a study of 51,603 nurses, those who drank one or more sodas a day (basically high-fructose corn syrup and carbonated water) gained more weight than those who consumed one or fewer a week, and faced greater risk for developing diabetes.[27] In another study, children who drank one extra soft drink a day had a 60 percent greater chance of becoming obese.[28] (Additional studies have also linked high-fructose corn syrup to other maladies, too, including that not-so-pleasant illness known as irritable bowel syndrome.)[29]

Trans Fats: It's What's for Dinner

Developed in the 1940s, trans fats (or trans fatty acids, if you'd like to get long-winded about it) come from vegetable oil that has been hydrogenated, converting unsaturated fatty acids into saturated ones. In processed foods, trans fats replace naturally occurring solid fats like butter and liquid oils.

Why does industry love trans fats? Because with them baked goods—cookies, cakes, crackers, even some bread—can sit on shelves longer. The other winning element: they're cheaper than other fats traditionally used in baking, such as butter or lard. With industry pushing it, by the 1960s, trans fats had become widely used in baked products and fast foods.[30]

Unfortunately, trans fats have some unwelcome side effects: They lower "good" cholesterol and increase the "bad," which in turn increases insulin resistance (elevating the risk of Type 2 diabetes) and contributes to coronary heart disease—the number-one cause of death in the United States, afflicting 13 million Americans per year.[31]

In 1994, Dr. Walter Willett and others from the Harvard School of Public Health estimated that thirty thousand premature deaths from coronary heart disease could be attributed to consuming trans fatty acids.[32]

Food industry representatives were on the case. They sponsored a review of the research, which concluded the following year that the "evidence was insufficient to take action"; more studies were needed.[33] Well, the Harvard researchers completed more research. In 1999 they upped the estimate to 100,000 deaths annually that could be prevented, just by reducing trans fat consumption.[34]

THE GIRTH OF A NATION

"Fast food kills more people in our community than crack," Michael Hurwitz says at the beginning of workshops on health with community members in the predominantly black and Latino neighborhood of Red Hook, Brooklyn, where he cofounded Added Value, a farm and education center. Those are shocking words, but tragically, true.

This radical experiment has hit low-income neighborhoods and communities of color hardest, with rates of Type 2 diabetes two to six times greater among African-Americans, Hispanics, and Native Americans than the non-Hispanic white population and obesity afflicting roughly one-third of African-American and Mexican-American women compared with one-fifth of white women.[35] Some of the poorest states in the union have the highest rates of obesity: Alabama and Mississippi, among the top ten poorest, rank number one and two in rates of obesity, with more than one in four obese adults.[36]

The epidemic is hitting children, too. When I was a kid, I didn't have many classmates who were overweight, and none I can remember who were obese. Today, childhood obesity is nearing 17 percent, more than triple what it was in 1975.[37] Research suggests that childhood obesity rates like these could mean a reduction of life expectancy by two to five years—equivalent to the impact of all cancers in the United States.[38] We also know that obese children are more prone to depression: One study found obese kids as likely to be depressed as kids undergoing chemotherapy for cancer.[39]

Obesity increases our chances of developing a range of illnesses, including hypertension, Type 2 diabetes, coronary heart disease, stroke, gallbladder disease, osteoarthritis, sleep apnea, respiratory problems, and some cancers, such as breast, colon, and prostate.[40] The Centers for Disease Control estimate that hundreds of thousands die annually from obesity-related illnesses,[41] and as many as 100 million American adults suffer from diet-related hypertension or pre-hypertension.[42]

These illnesses and swelling obesity in essentially one generation cannot be explained away simply by too many hours on the couch watching *American Idol*. No, it's the food: our diet is largely to blame for the obesity epidemic, as it is for the increase in certain cancers and hormonal and neurological disorders associated with exposure to toxins in our food and environment, agricultural chemicals chief among them.

—⁓—

The futuristic world Woody Allen dreamed up in *Sleeper* included not only those incredulous doctors, but also a farm with larger-than-human bananas and tomatoes. A prescient nod to genetically modified foods? Maybe, but Allen probably could never have fathomed what would actually happen to our farmland: how diversified small farms would give way to industrial factories-in-the-field where toxic chemicals and wasteful use of water and petroleum would drive production. Nor could he have predicted the effects of the diet of the future (*our* diet, that is) on the human body. Or, maybe he could have—it just wouldn't have been that funny.

THREE

Ordering the Wake-Up Call

S o if we're being sickened by the food we eat and how it's grown, why aren't more of us guinea pigs storming the barricades? Why don't more of us see through the six illusions? To answer these questions, we need to first remind ourselves how much is riding on our not ordering the wake-up call, on our swallowing this great experiment and its grand illusions.

When you combine the annual sales of the top ten biggest seed and agrochemical companies, food manufacturers and traders, and food retailers, you find they brought in nearly $1 trillion in 2002.[1] The top ten farm chemical companies alone have annual sales of more than $22 billion.[2] The fast-food and restaurant industry also brings home billions every year. In 2004, McDonald's raked in $19 billion.[3] If your head is spinning with all these *b*'s, *t*'s, and triple-digit zeroes, just remember: we're talking about a lot of money, with the biggest food companies boasting revenues that rival some nations' GDPs.

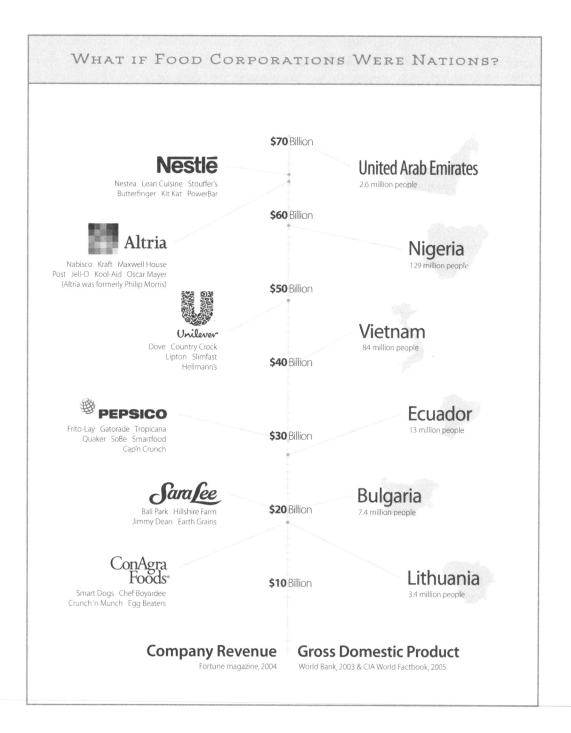

WHAT IF FOOD CORPORATIONS WERE NATIONS?

$70 Billion

Nestlé
Nestea   Lean Cuisine   Stouffer's
Butterfinger   Kit Kat   PowerBar

United Arab Emirates
2.6 million people

$60 Billion

Altria
Nabisco   Kraft   Maxwell House
Post   Jell-O   Kool-Aid   Oscar Mayer
(Altria was formerly Philip Morris)

Nigeria
129 million people

$50 Billion

Unilever
Dove   Country Crock
Lipton   Slimfast
Hellmann's

Vietnam
84 million people

$40 Billion

PEPSICO
Frito-Lay   Gatorade   Tropicana
Quaker   SoBe   Smartfood
Cap'n Crunch

Ecuador
13 million people

$30 Billion

SaraLee
Ball Park   Hillshire Farm
Jimmy Dean   Earth Grains

Bulgaria
7.4 million people

$20 Billion

ConAgra Foods®
Smart Dogs   Chef Boyardee
Crunch'n Munch   Egg Beaters

Lithuania
3.4 million people

$10 Billion

Company Revenue
Fortune magazine, 2004

Gross Domestic Product
World Bank, 2003 & CIA World Factbook, 2005

Don't Touch That Dial:
Advertising and Our Psyche

Through overt advertising and harder-to-perceive public relations campaigns and front groups, through political contributions, lobbying and influencing government agencies, the food and agrichemical industries have been shaping and controlling policy for quite a while now. These policies in turn shape our access to Grub, the health of our environment, and ultimately our bodies.

Every day we're bombarded with sales pitches for food products—ads in subways, elevators, in the eighteen minutes of commercials per hour on television, even on bathroom stalls.[4] Many even infuse textbooks and line the shelves of our bookstores. Preschool and kindergarten children can now study math with the *M&M's Brand Chocolate Candies Counting Book* or curl up at night with their parents and read *The Cheerios Christmas Play Book.*

It shouldn't surprise us that we're so inundated. The food industry is one of the top advertisers in the United States, and the United States outspends the world.[5] Globally, dollars spent on advertising are predicted to surpass half a trillion in 2005; half of that will be by U.S. companies.[6] McDonald's alone spends over $1 billion every year.[7] (This is not money these companies pull from the ether. We pay for it every time we buy their products.) In contrast, the entire federal nutrition education budget amounts to just one-fifth of the advertising budget for Altoids mints.[8]

While even the most astute media consumers may think themselves immune to the manipulation of ads, new science is showing that our minds may be more vulnerable than we might like to believe. Using MRI scans of the human brain, Baylor College of Medicine neuroscientist Read Montague discovered that when he administered blind taste-tests of Coke and Pepsi, Pepsi came out on top. But when the same subjects drank the sodas with the brands exposed, they chose Coke. Montague observed that during the blind tests the area of the brain that processes feelings of reward became more excited. With the brands revealed, the area associated with cognitive powers such as memory of prior impressions kicked in. It seems "brand influence" can override even our taste buds.[9]

Advertisers are constantly seeking new ways to insert their message—and their brand—into our psyche. In an attempt to align their diet with healthy eating, Atkins Nutritionals, Inc. released the "Sensible Approach" food pyramid. It looks nearly identical to the former USDA-approved one, but unlike the government version, this one's quadrants are filled with Atkins fare. Trying to get in good with hip-hop culture, McDonald's offered cash to rappers who refer to "Big Mac" in a hit song.[10] "McDonald's retains final approval of the lyrics," *Advertising Age* explained.[11] I guess singers riffing off the fact that one Big Mac hits you with 60 percent of your recommended maximum daily dose of saturated fats and one-third of your salt wouldn't go over too well with Mickey D execs.

Kids are the most vulnerable to this kind of spin—and advertising in general. That's why several European countries ban advertising to children. Ireland bans television commercials for fast food. Sweden, Norway, Austria, and Luxembourg ban all television advertising geared toward children flat out.[12]

By contrast, kids in the United States are pummeled with junk food and beverage advertising from day one: even some baby bottles now sport corporate logos.[13] Food and beverage marketing to kids in the United States eats up between $10 and $12 billion a year—enough to provide health insurance for every uninsured kid in the country.[14] On television alone, the average child is hit with tens of thousands of food advertisements every year, the vast majority of them for unhealthy, highly sweetened foods.[15] (When was the last time you saw an advertisement for green beans on Saturday morning cartoons?)

When restrictions on advertising to kids were proposed in the United States in 2005, companies like General Mills, Kellogg, and Kraft Foods teamed up with advertising associations to form the Alliance for American Advertising.[16] Its goal? To "beat back the public perception that advertising makes children obese."[17] They're right about one thing: it's not the advertising that makes kids obese; it's the food being advertised that does.

But "advertising" happens in subtle ways, too. Consider the article "Soft Drinks, Childhood Overweight, and the Role of Nutrition Educators: Let's Base Our Solutions on Reality and Sound Science," published in the *Journal of Nutrition Education and Behavior,* denying the claims that soda is so bad for you.[18] The article was written with funding from the Coca-Cola Company. Just a year before, the company's foundation had given $1 million to the American Academy of Pediatric Dentistry.[19] Don't worry, drink up, kids!

When the American Dietetic Association, the nation's largest organization of food and nutrition professionals, meets every year, its educational workshops are dotted with sponsors you'd recognize. Among the workshops in 2004 were "A Spoonful of Novel Nutrients Helps the Medicine Go Down," sponsored by Novartis Medical Nutrition; "Naturally Nutrient Rich Foods: Packing More Power on Your Plate," sponsored by the National Cattlemen's Beef Association and Cattlemen's Beef Board; and "Update on Dairy Nutrition and Health: Research to Recommendations," sponsored by the National Dairy Council. Along with these workshops, food companies (whose products are often of dubious health value) sponsor other conference features from conference bags (the sugar substitute Equal) to hotel room keys (the diet supplement drink Ensure) to hotel "room drops" where companies pay to have promotional goodies placed in attendees' rooms (Heinz, Kraft Foods/Nabisco).

THE TRUTH, THE WHOLE TRUTH, AND NOTHING BUT THE TRUTH: THINK TANKS, FRONT GROUPS, AND SPIN

Legendary Hollywood film producer Robert Evans was famous for saying "There are three sides to every story: Your side, my side, and the truth. And no one is lying." Well, that may be true in Evans's Hollywood, but in real life there may be different sides to a story, and one side may certainly be lying . . . or at least not telling the whole truth.

I wonder what Evans would make of this story. On March 7, 2005, the Center for Global Food Issues posted an online article that stated. "Environmental activists claim that synthetic fertilizer from farms is threatening the marine life in the Gulf of Mexico by causing the rampant spread of a 'dead zone' of low-oxygen water." The article denied any connection between this dead zone and agricultural chemical runoff: "New research . . . shows that the Gulf of Mexico had the seasonal 'dead zones' . . . as early as 1817—long before farmers even settled the Mississippi Valley."[20]

That same week, one of the world's most authoritative science journals, *Nature*, published a peer-reviewed study from Stanford University researchers with a different take.

"Inarguably, the effects of marine nitrogen pollution are becoming extremely widespread and severe as a consequence of the global expansion of industrialized agriculture and the intensification of certain practices," noted the researchers. "Nitrogen-based fertilizers are the primary source of [this] pollution."[21]

"I looked at five years of satellite data and found a direct correspondence between the use of nitrogen fertilizers and algal blooms," explained a lead author on the study. "These blooms represent millions of microscopic weeds in the ocean like a fish tank that hasn't been cleaned. In the ocean these blooms can be toxic, generating the low-oxygen dead zones."[22]

Five years of satellite data is pretty compelling. Top-notch researchers and peer-reviewed research seem pretty trustworthy. And the Center for Global Food Issues? It is a project of the Hudson Institute, a think tank funded in part by agribusiness giants such as Archer Daniels Midland, ConAgra Foods, Monsanto, and Novartis.[23]

The Center's director, and the author of the article, Dennis T. Avery, is a vocal proponent of chemical farming and critic of organic practices. His book *Saving the Planet with Pesticides and Plastic* rejects claims that farm chemicals harm the environment or our health. He disputes, for instance, the widely accepted—and factually proven—human and environmental toll of the infamous Agent Orange, code name for the herbicide sprayed by the U.S. military over 3.6 million acres of Vietnam during the war there.[24] Avery quotes journalist Jon Franklin, who stated "the squadron that sprayed Agent Orange . . . wore boxer shorts and tennis shoes, and were commonly covered with [it] . . . Well . . . their health, ten and fifteen years after exposure, was very normal. No excess cancer, heart disease, alcoholism."[25]

But scientific studies have long shown the link between Agent Orange and serious illnesses. Vietnamese scientists have linked the herbicide to upwards of 150,000 birth defects and nearly 1 million other illnesses in their country.[26] An Institute of Medicine committee investigating the health effects of the herbicide on U.S. veterans has determined that exposure can be associated with certain cancers, including a particularly deadly form of leukemia, as well as other serious health problems and birth defects in the children of exposed vets.[27] In a 1984 landmark class-action lawsuit, seven American chemical companies agreed to a settlement of $180 million with 291,000 veterans exposed to Agent Orange in the war.[28]

Avery's counterevidence? As I said, he seals his case with one anecdote from one journalist.

And what about Avery's dismissal of the connection between farm chemicals and the dead zone? While he is partly correct—algal blooms can appear naturally—Avery misleads us by ignoring the *whole* story. We may have had algal blooms for centuries, but nothing close to the scale we witness now. Today, the dead zone in the Gulf of Mexico swells each summer to the size of New Jersey, thanks in part to more than 1 million tons of fertilizers and agricultural waste that run off from farms and wash down the Mississippi every year.[29] Dead zones in our oceans are so concerning that the United Nations ranked them as one of the greatest threats to the global environment.[30]

Now, maybe Avery doesn't read *Nature* magazine, or track United Nations warnings, or consult scholars with expertise in the fields he comments on, but I find it more likely that his ignorance of the evidence is an intentional disregard for the whole truth.

There's a reason why when you take the stand you swear to tell the truth, the whole truth, and nothing but the truth. A partial truth may be just as misleading as a lie, or even more so. After all, partial truths are harder to refute than bald-faced lies.

The partial truth can be particularly misleading when packaged with an air of objectivity. Avery, for instance, is head of the Center for Global Food Issues, which sounds nonpartisan and fair-minded. But his center, based out of the Hudson Institute, is just one of numerous industry-funded think tanks that conceal their bias behind a veneer of objectivity.

"Powerful corporate interests have learned to hide behind front groups with noble sounding names such as the American Council on Science and Health, the Harvard Center for Risk Analysis, and the Center for Consumer Freedom," says media analyst John Stauber, coauthor of *Trust Us, We're Experts!* (Consider the euphemistic name-changing of CropLife America. It was formerly known as the American Crop Protection Association, and was founded, in 1933, as the National Agricultural Chemicals Association.)

"These front groups claim the mantle of the public interest, but their agenda dovetails with that of their corporate funders, and they try to conceal the degree to which they are the creation of, or funded by, corporations and their lobbyists," adds Stauber.

Front groups organize briefings on Capitol Hill, publish articles and op-eds, issue press releases, write books. They infiltrate professional associations; they go on talk shows. And they build websites. Think you can pick out a front group from the real deal? Try this one.

FoodSecurity.net is just one URL extension away from FoodSecurity.org, but it is worlds apart. The Food Security Network (the .net) says it is "an independent, non-profit coalition of people throughout the world dedicated to participating in an open, informed and impactful dialogue addressing solutions to global food security concerns through sustainable agricultural practices." But a little sleuthing exposes a different identity entirely.

FoodSecurity.net is registered to Graydon Forrer, the managing director of Life Sciences Strategies LLC, which specializes in communications for bioscience companies.[31] When he registered the website in 1999, Forrer was director of executive communications at Monsanto.[32] He is also an outspoken critic of organic food and farming, appearing, for instance, with Alex Avery (son and colleague of Dennis Avery) at a 2001 conference about agricultural biotechnology on a panel called "Fear-Based Marketing by Organic Retailers: A Major Factor Driving Anti-Biotechnology Public Opinion."[33]

Investigative journalists did some digging and found that the few posts on the Food Security.net website were from some interesting people and places, including e-mail addresses that could be traced to bivwood.com, the website for the Bivings Group, a strategic communications firm that has represented Monsanto, and from someone named Andura Smetacek.[34] Presumably the same Andura Smetacek (how many can there be?) who posted online criticisms in 2001 of a UC Berkeley professor and graduate student whose article in *Nature* that year raised concerns about the contamination of local varieties of corn in Mexico with genetically modified corn from the United States.[35] Smetacek's allegations swept across the Internet and online discussion groups. Though unfounded, they added to an industry-backed campaign to discredit the research.[36]

And who is Smetacek? Turns out, Smetacek is a *nom-de-email,* an online persona created by a biotech public relations firm.[37]

"Sometimes only the client knows the precise role we played," Bivings likes to boast, according to British journalist George Monbiot, who covered the story.[38] "Sometimes, in other words, real people have no idea that they are being managed by fake ones," quips Monbiot.[39]

The Forrer and Monsanto connections, the Smetacek and Bivings posts, and the lack of any substantive content on the site, all suggest that FoodSecurity.net is probably not a "coalition of people throughout the world dedicated to participating in an open, informed and impactful dialogue." And what about FoodSecurity.org? If you want to know for sure, dig for yourself: find out about their members, their funders, their board of directors. If you do, you'll find, well, it really *is* a coalition of organizations and communities that really are working to address hunger and access to healthy foods.

DIALING FOR DOLLARS

Sometimes shaping our understanding of key issues and public policy doesn't require creating a fictitious organization. It just requires supporting the right people, the right ways, at the right time, and using lobbying muscle when necessary.

In recent years lobbying on Capitol Hill has become a booming business, a $2.1 billion dollar a year business, to be exact, with food- and agriculture-specific lobbying accounting for $51 million of the total in 2004.[40] But the official figures tend to underestimate the *real* totals, since firms often report their spending late—sometimes many years late—or, never. Although it's required by law to report your lobbying spending, one study found that over a six-year period 20 percent of lobbying forms were never filed.[41] The 2004 food-related lobbying total also doesn't account for the $13.2 million spent that year by Altria Group (formerly Philip Morris), which owns food giant Kraft. Nor does it count the $26.3 million spent on lobbying by the chemical industry, whose interests include farm chemicals, too.

Contributions to political campaigns, through individuals giving directly to candidates or to political action committees, are another way industry influences politics. That same year, employees of agribusiness companies directed an additional $52.7 million to political campaigns through individual donations or PACs, nearly three-quarters of it to Republicans.[42]

In other words, beyond their budgets for advertising, public relations, and other media, the food industry and their employees spent at least $105 million on political influence during just one year. (Oops, I didn't mean agribusiness spent it; we did—when we bought their food products.)

Why the willingness to pay such big bucks? One answer is that it's a pretty good return on investment. Among other rewards, agribusiness was guaranteed in the 2002 Farm Bill $180 billion in federal subsidies over ten years, a $73.5 billion increase over existing programs.[43] These subsidies were maintained despite a huge federal deficit and complaints from nations around the world that our subsidies violate international trade agreements by providing unfair advantage to big agricultural companies in the United States.

Trolling through the U.S. Office of Public Records online, you can uncover details about where a chunk of your food dollar goes.

Monsanto, for instance, reported spending $3.3 million on lobbying in 2004.[44] With their "specific lobbying issues" described as "All legislation regulation affecting the manufacture of agriculture products, specialty chemical products, food products generally and specifically."[45]

The Biotechnology Industry Organization (BIO), formed in 1993 to represent companies in the emerging fields of medical and agricultural biotech, spent $5.2 million in 2004 on lobbying, three times as much as they had in 1998.[46] This money was devoted to lobbying for bills like HR 4651 to "establish a Federal interagency task force to promote the benefits, safety, and potential uses of agricultural biotechnology outside the United States."[47] In other words, the bill would appropriate taxpayer dollars to promote genetically modified foods overseas. No wonder BIO is gunning for it—taxpayers would help underwrite their members' marketing.

The Grocery Manufacturers of America (GMA) is another trade group that pools the money of its members—among the world's largest food and beverage companies—to lobby every year on their behalf.[48] Along with congressional testimonies and public relations campaigns and more than a million dollars a year for lobbying, GMA keeps busy writing a lot of letters.[49]

From January 2003 to February 2005, GMA wrote more than two dozen "letters of opposition" to bills proposed in sixteen states that would promote childhood nutrition and limit or ban junk food in schools.[50] To the state of Oklahoma, the GMA wrote: "Restrictions such as those suggested in SB 265 for the sake of solving obesity *would do nothing* to motivate students, parents, or communities to take the steps necessary to improve their overall health."[51] (emphasis added)

It wouldn't? Decide for yourself: the bill proposes eliminating "access to sugary drinks and snacks; except for special occasions" in elementary schools; requiring "only healthy choices be accessible during the day" in middle schools; and that "healthy choices (snacks and beverages that meet USDA guidelines)" be offered in the state's high schools.[52] Sounds pretty reasonable to me. (Despite GMA efforts, some of the biggest school districts in the country *have* banned sodas in schools, and a number of states are pursuing statewide policies.)

These trade associations also wield their influence to shape what gets said and done, or not said and not done, on Capitol Hill. In 2002, the EPA Office of Prevention, Pesticides, and Toxic Substances received a letter of complaint from CropLife America and Responsible Industry for a Sound Environment (RISE) a few months before an EPA-sponsored forum on pesticides.[53] The letter complained that the forum would "malign or discourage the use of pesticides," naming three participants who "have a clear record of such practice." The "program, as planned, will simply become yet another 'Officially Sponsored' opportunity to bash pesticides and achieve political agendas," asserted the letter. The offending presentations included such incendiary talks as "Pesticides and Children" and "Pesticide Usage, Health Effects, and Populations at Risk."[54]

CropLife America members, as I've noted, include virtually all U.S. agriculture chemical and biotechnology companies. RISE is a lobbying and public relations trade organization for the pesticide and fertilizer industry. (They share offices in D.C.)[55]

The forum was postponed ten months. When it was held, the contested experts were not on the agenda.[56]

THE CLUB FACTOR

Anyone can find lobbying records, even front groups can be uncovered with a little detective work. Not as apparent, though, is the huge effect on our lives of what happens when a relatively small group of people move between top agribusiness positions and the think tanks that influence policy, between the lobbying and law firms that defend the food industry and the government agencies that regulate it.

When the authors of *Toxic Deception* investigated this "revolving door" in the chemical industry, here's what they found: Of nearly 350 lobbyists and lawyers who worked from 1990 to 1995 for the chemical companies and trade associations they researched, nearly half had previously worked for federal departments or agencies, or in congressional offices.[57] And they found nearly half of EPA officials who left top-level jobs in toxics and pesticides from 1980 to 1995 went on to work for chemical companies, their lobbying firms, or their trade associations.[58] All told, since 1998, 2,200 lobbyists (and counting) have also worked inside government—from members of Congress to high-level positions at the USDA, EPA, and more.[59]

Consider a few examples when it comes to our food, such as Michael Taylor's circular path. When he left the Food and Drug Administration, Taylor joined a law firm representing Monsanto, after which he returned to the FDA, where he helped set standards for biotech food. He later joined Monsanto as vice president for public policy.[60]

Or Dan Glickman's professional trajectory: when Glickman left his post as USDA Secretary in 2001, he joined a D.C. law firm that advises its corporate clients on policy, including food safety and biotechnology.[61] Or Ann Veneman's: when she was appointed to head the USDA in 2001, she brought with her longstanding ties to agribusiness, both as a former director of the biotech company Calgene (now owned by Monsanto) and as a member of a policy council funded by agribusiness giants Cargill, Nestlé, Kraft, and Archer Daniels Midland, among others.[62]

Now there is nothing necessarily illegal about any of this, but the more this revolving door turns the more the line is blurred between those working in *our* interest and those getting paid to work in *industry's.* As the same people move in and out of public and private roles, they foster a sort of club—a relatively exclusive and tight-knit one. It's a club in which the reigning assumption is that what's best for industry is best for all of us and where innovative ideas, critical reflection, and the challenging of orthodoxies rarely occur. All of which may help explain why some of its members didn't seem too interested in talking with people like me.

Though months before their annual meeting CropLife America had approved my attendance, just days before I was to leave an e-mail citing company policy informed me I was no longer allowed to attend. With my travel and hotel already booked, I went anyway. When I arrived at the registration table, CropLife president Jay Vroom said, "We've read some of your stuff on the Web and we understand that your position . . . may not be in accord with where we are coming from, but we'd like to have a dialogue rather than saying we'd like to pretend you don't exist."

Hmm, I wasn't exactly getting the "dialogue" vibe when I was told not to come to the conference. His version of "dialogue"? He permitted me to attend one conference session with the EPA's Stephen Johnson, but not other presentations by representatives of such presumably public institutions as the World Trade Organization.

When I tried to reach a Syngenta communications officer with questions about atrazine (one of the most widely used herbicides in the country), it took multiple phone calls, five months, and eight e-mails before I got a response to my basic questions.

I even got the cold shoulder from a professor at a public university who had spoken at an American Chemical Society conference. When I inquired about his presentation refuting research about the benefits of organic food, he e-mailed back with these five words: "Sorry, I can't help you." When I tried to make it easier, asking if there were any published records of his talk or research papers on which he based his remarks, he e-mailed back: "No, there aren't any."

At the 2005 Biotechnology Industry Organization's annual conference, the Pennsylvania National Conventional Center was teeming with more than 18,000 people, including representatives from biotech companies, academic institutes, and state biotechnology centers in fifty-six countries.[63] At a session called "Organic and Biotech: Won't You Be My Neighbor?" the four panelists all concurred that genetically modified foods pose no dangers to public health or the environment and organic agriculture. When one attendee went so far as to suggest that opponents of biotech foods should be tried for "crimes against humanity," no one objected. No one even hinted at the counterevidence from reputable scientists about the contamination of organic fields with genetically modified organisms and other concerns with the technology.[64]

During the Q&A, I asked if GMOs posed no environmental risk why a company like Monsanto would bribe Indonesian government officials to bypass environmental safety testing of biotech crops that Monsanto sought to introduce there, as the company had in 2005. The panelists shrugged. An audience member shouted: "Because that's the only way you get things done there!"

As I was leaving the session, the BIO communications director quickly approached me. My question was very "off topic" and was a "very weird question to ask," she said. "I'm wondering why you're here," she added, saying this was an industry conference and that she knew most of the journalists there, but didn't know me. (She then asked for my conference pass.)

The media present included journalists from the *New York Times, Business Week,* and the *Wall Street Journal,* among others. But by "industry conference," she seemed to imply that no one was expected to raise challenging questions. In the roomful of more than 150 people, no one had. Off topic? Maybe by off topic she just meant "off message."

These are just a few examples of how industry shuts out public inquiry, but they have other means of blocking our hearing information that might shatter the illusions and uncover the great American experiment. Increasingly in recent years, industry has targeted scientists and journalists whose research has raised questions about agricultural chemicals and biotech food, attempting to discredit their research, strip them of their jobs, block their books, articles and reports, or destroy their reputations.[65] One incident hit close to home.

When my father wrote *Against the Grain* in the late 1990s with Britt Bailey, their research disproved many of the claims of biotech food proponents, including increased yields. In 1998, *Against the Grain* was headed for print when the publisher, Vital Health Publishing, received a threatening six-page letter from Monsanto lawyers. Though the lawyer had not seen the manuscript, the letter raised the concern that the book would disparage the company's herbicide Roundup. With concern about the cost of defending themselves against Monsanto, the publisher balked. Though my father and Bailey eventually found the appropriately named Common Courage Press to release the book, their experience makes me wonder how many other books may never have seen the light of day.[66]

In 1972, the American psychologist Irving Janis came up with a way to explain what this club factor does to decision making. With a wink to Orwell, Janis called it "groupthink." It's what happens when a group's disregard for conflicting evidence and desire for unanimity overcome rational thinking. Among the consequences? Alternative choices are not explored and risks aren't fully examined. Once a decision is made there is no reassessment, and really smart groups of people make terrible—sometimes fatal—decisions. Janis used groupthink to explain such debacles as the Bay of Pigs and the invasion of Vietnam.[67]

Maybe the pesticide and food industry club factor is fostering just what Janis feared: locking even the brightest minds onto terribly dangerous paths—for all of us.

Guinea Pigs of the World, Unite!

Eating is the most essential act of every living creature. And in virtually every human culture, growing, eating, and sharing food has a spiritual dimension, too. Today, eating is also unquestionably a political act. Our food choices, conscious or not, shape our world.

Tapping our common sense, we can wrest control of these choices from the advertisers and marketers, from the salesmen and chemical hawkers. For despite the spin and the lobbying, the advertising and the corporate propaganda, the truth about what's healthy is really quite simple. Indeed, it is right in front of our noses. As my grandmother would have said, "If it were a snake, it would have bitten you."

And what a happy coincidence: choosing Grub—making the most common sense choices about our food—improves our own health and that of the planet, farmers, and farmworkers, all at the same time.

Choosing Grub may just mean that within our lifetime we'll be able to look back at this strange and failed American food experiment with the same incredulity with which we look back on that doctor who suggested cigarettes to my grandmother. It will seem—and be—just that odd. Food will no longer be a source of illness and unhappiness, what little "conventional" produce remains will be labeled "grown with chemicals," and funding for sustainable farming will surpass that for the newest chemical cocktail or genetically modified twist.

While we're striving for this day, we can improve our own health and limit our own exposure to toxins through our food choices and our support of stricter standards. Exactly what those CropLife execs don't want us to do; it might make their paying for a weekend at the Ritz-Carlton a little trickier.

Guinea pigs of the world, unite! We have nothing to lose but waste, pollution, illness, environmental devastation . . . and our love handles.

Part

TWO

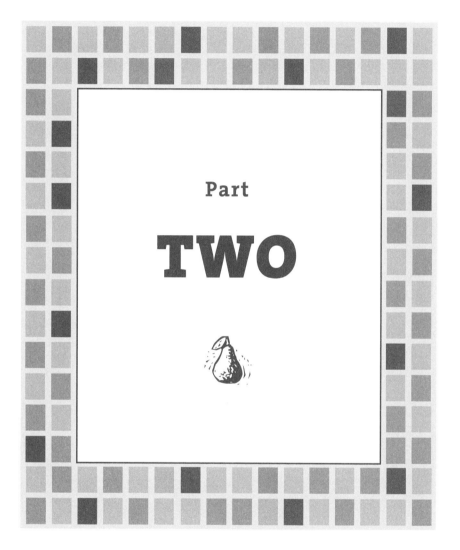

FOUR

Grub 101

GUINEA PIGS AT THE BARRICADES

I am sitting on a plane on the tarmac in St. Louis, Missouri—not the first place you'd imagine I'd be sensing the emergence of Grub, but that's exactly what I'm feeling. Yesterday, on a muggy day in June, I spoke at a conference sponsored by the Sierra Club in Godfrey, Illinois, where I met dozens of people from towns along the banks of the Mississippi and Illinois rivers asking fundamental questions about food. In a region hit hard by deindustrialization, they are working to create innovative strategies to ensure their community has access to organic and sustainably raised whole foods, grown locally and from companies and farms with fair workplace practices. They are, in a word, bringing Grub to life.

The folks I met in Godfrey are no anomaly. Across the country, from college campuses in Missoula, Montana, to rural Pennsylvania, from neighborhoods in Seattle to the southside of Chicago, students, farmers, activists, policymakers, parents, teachers, and more are living proof that the guinea pigs may just be storming the barricades after all.

For alongside the not-so-great American experiment and the unhealthy and destructive food system described in Part One, another trend has been emerging.

I saw it in Godfrey: I saw it in the organic farmer from La Vista Community Supported

Garden; in the schoolteacher supporting the children-oriented Discovery garden; in the representative from the local food crisis center. I tasted it in the food from Biver's Farm, New Roots CSA, and the local farmers' market.

Yes, in Godfrey I caught another glimpse of the three interlocking elements bringing to life what we call Grub: the revolution in ecological farming, the revival of local foods, and the flourishing of food justice.

Evidence of these trends is popping up all around us. To believe me, though, you have to expand your mind to hold the "both/and." In Part One, you read how burdened we are by the costs of what journalist Eric Schlosser calls the "dark side of the all-American meal." You read about damage done by a food system based on highest return to shareholder, not on the principles of good health, or of democracy.

Yes, but . . . that is only half the story.

Over the past generation, and picking up pace in the past ten years, a counterrevolution has been blossoming. You don't see it advertised on billboards, or broadcast too often on the nightly news, but across the country millions are choosing the sustainable, just foods we call Grub.

While many may still be reaching for the prescriptions of the latest fad diet or drastic surgery, many others, like the folks in Godfrey, are embracing a healthier relationship to food, and making the connections between their dietary choices and our world. You can see it in the majority of Americans who say they're concerned about the chemicals used to grow their food; in the millions choosing locally grown and certified "fair trade" food; in the nearly half of Americans who say they've bought organics recently.[1]

These food choices are not a diet, per se, at least not in the way most of us think about diets. Choosing Grub is not a get-thin-quick instruction guide. (Though eating this way may reduce your waistline as you get in tune with your natural tastes, hungers, and desires, unmanipulated by high-paid advertising execs; it did mine.) Making these food choices is not a holier-than-thou prescription, or an inflexible commandment. For nothing is more personal than what we choose to eat. No, Grub is a set of choices we each can make that will radically transform our personal lives, communities, and our world.

That might sound like hyperbole, but read on.

Here in Part Two, you'll learn about the three pillars of Grub, demystifying the jargon about what this food is and arming you with the tools to wade through information about the benefits of these choices.

Consider Grub inspiring ideas for a way of eating—a way to make choices—that are healthy for our bodies as well as our communities. As you make these choices, you'll be joining the millions of us at the barricades, transforming our bodies, our lives, and the world.

Welcome to the frontlines.

PILLAR 1: THE ECOLOGICAL FARMING REVOLUTION

In the past thirty years, organic foods have moved out of the patchouli-scented aisles of food coops into the fluorescent-lit grocery stores of Main Street America, or more accurately (because not too many Main Streets remain) into the Wal-Marts, Costcos, and Sam's Clubs of the new millennium.[2] Organic products are the fastest growing area of the food industry, increasing 20 to 25 percent every year since 1990.[3] Compare these figures with an essentially stagnant food industry and you really start to see the significance.

Thirty years ago, organic foods might have meant "you had to chew more," as Gary Hirshberg, the CEO of one of the largest organic dairy companies, likes to put it. But today it's haute cuisine. Even hoity-toity *Vogue* magazine has featured the grand dame of organics, chef and restaurateur Alice Waters. And vegetarianism, once more associated with yurt dwellers than Golden Arches connoisseurs, is now seen as pedestrian: McDonald's serves up veggie burgers.

Despite these strides, looking at the actual share of organic farmland in the United States is a bit of a buzz-kill: less than half of 1 percent (0.4 percent, to be exact) of all U.S. cropland and a measly 0.1 percent of all pastureland was organic in 2003.[4] Organic production levels are slightly better for specialty crops, but at most we're usually only talking about up to 5 percent.[5] Overall, of roughly 2 million farmers in the United States, only 18,000 are raising certified organic products.[6]

In a country that prides itself on being a world leader, we're definitely behind the curve. Most of the 108 countries using certified organic farming practices have significantly higher percentages of organic production than we do.[7] Italy, roughly the size of Arizona, has nearly five times as many organic farmers as the United States. Proportionally, Italy devotes 100 times more of its farmland to organic production than the United States does.[8] Though the introduction of the USDA organic certification in 2002 has significantly increased the demand for and awareness of organics, we certainly have a long way to go.

When some people think of "organic," they still conjure images of throwback farmers,

Luddites forgoing the benefits of chemicals for a Pollyanna vision of an idealized agrarian past. To those with that attitude, science and organics certainly don't go hand in hand.

But organic farming today, using methods that promote soil health and natural and biological pest management and that eschew most manmade chemicals, is based on a more sophisticated and nuanced understanding of biology and ecology than is industrial agriculture.

These ecological farming practices have evolved since the 1940s and prove to yield more, be more sustainable, and use markedly fewer nonrenewable resources than chemical farming. They are a manifestation of the other significant revolution in agriculture in the past century: yes, there was the post–World War II chemical revolution, the hybrid-seed and farm chemical Green Revolution, and its turn-of-the-century redux the Gene Revolution, but there has also been a much less reported, but possibly even more astounding, ecological revolution in farming.

When agriculture's chemical age was born after World War II, it also gave rise to innovators who believed another path was possible, one that wasn't dependent on chemicals and foreign oil. The founding fathers—and mothers!—of this movement include Austrian-born Rudolf Steiner, who introduced a spiritual dimension to organic farming in the 1920s, seeing the soil as part of a living sentient system; Lady Eve Balfour, a founder of the British Soil Association, who initiated the first ecological research project on her farm in 1939 (the Haughley Experiment, as it was called, would continue for another three decades); and J. I. Rodale, who helped bring organic farming to the United States in the 1940s, and whose work emphasized the importance of soil health. As Balfour said in a 1977 speech, the early twentieth-century organic pioneers "all succeeded in breaking away from the narrow confines of the preconceived ideas that dominated the scientific thinking of their day." They broke new ground with strategies to produce high yields without the risks of chemicals, the water wasted, the topsoil lost, or the nonrenewable resources used up.

Since those early organic pioneers, innovators in the field have seen the higher yields and other benefits of organic farming go beyond their wildest dreams.[9] In the largest study of its kind, researchers examined 200 sustainable agriculture projects in 52 countries covering roughly 70 million acres. The conclusion? Sustainable practices can "lead to substantial increases" in production, with some farmers realizing yield increases as great as 150 percent.[10]

In one of the longest-running studies comparing organic and chemically grown soybeans and corn in the United States, researchers found that organic techniques not only produced comparable yields, but also used on average 30 percent less fossil energy, while reducing soil erosion and conserving water.[11] The organic crops also absorbed and retained more carbon in the soil.[12] Why is that so important? Because retaining the carbon helps reduce carbon dioxide in the atmosphere, one of the greenhouse gases that contributes to global warming (or, as it might more appropriately be called, climate chaos).

Organic farming might benefit us in the near future for another reason: organic farming creates plants that are more resilient to droughts and floods, attributes that will only become more valuable as global climate chaos worsens.[13]

Though GMO proponents tout *their* technology—not organic farming—as a way to increase production while decreasing pesticide use, the opposite seems to be true. An extensive study of GMO soy found significantly lower yields than comparable non-GMO varieties[14] and a nine-year review of GMOs and pesticides found that the production of genetically modified corn, soybeans, and cotton has led to an overall increase in pesticide use.[15]

As organic farming evolved and production increased, pioneering organic farmers and their supportive eaters wanted a way to distinguish these products: a third-party certification with an identifiable seal so consumers could look at a label and trust the food.

By the late 1980s a patchwork of state certification programs had been created. But as the demand for organic foods increased, the need to create a national seal seemed imperative. And as large-scale farmers began to move into organic farming, the need to have a seal that would be internationally accepted also mounted. By 1990, an act in Congress sealed the deal: the USDA would create an official organic label. It would take another twelve contentious years before the guidelines would be finalized.

For most of us, genetically modified and irradiated foods and food grown on land treated with sewage sludge would not fit in with our gut sense of what "organic" is. But according to the initial USDA standards proposed in 1997, all of these foods would have been considered organic—would have, that is, if not for an uppity public.

Within days of releasing the proposed guidelines for public comment, the USDA was barraged with thousands of irate letters. Consumers also deluged their elected officials, who in turn put pressure on the USDA. All told, during the 180-day public comment period, 280,000 people voiced their opinions, more than the USDA had ever heard from on any issue to date, and a new national network—the Organic Consumers Association—was born to advocate for and amplify the voice of hundreds of thousands of concerned eaters.[16]

The USDA went back to the drawing board. Five years later, in October 2002, the agency announced its standards—all 554 pages of them. Now just a few years later, you can find the USDA organic label on foods in most supermarkets throughout this country. Here's how to decipher what the label means.

Deciphering the Organic Label

USDA Organic Definition: An ecological production management system that promotes and enhances biodiversity, biological cycles and soil biological activity. It is based on minimal use of off-farm inputs and on management practices that restore, maintain and enhance ecological harmony.

No organic ingredients can be processed with genetically modified organisms, irradiation, or sewage sludge. (See the chart on page 86 for differences between organic and nonorganic meat and dairy.)

"100% Organic" USDA ORGANIC	Products can contain only certified-organic ingredients (excluding water and salt). ▪ Can display the USDA organic logo and/or the certifying agent's logo and state 100% organic.
"Organic" USDA ORGANIC	95% of the ingredients must be certified organic (excluding water and salt). The remaining 5% must be nonorganic ingredients approved by the National Organic Standards Board or nonorganically produced agricultural products not commercially available in organic form. (A short list of approved nonorganically produced agricultural products includes: cornstarch, specific gums, kelp, lecithin, and a type of pectin.) ▪ Can display the USDA organic logo and/or another certifier's logo.
"Made with Organic Ingredients"	Must be made with at least 70% organic ingredients. ▪ Can display the certifier's logo, but *not* the USDA organic logo. Can list up to three of the organic ingredients on the front panel.
Organic ingredients listed on ingredient panel	Specific organic ingredients can be listed only on the ingredients panel. There are no restrictions on the other ingredients. ▪ *Cannot* display the USDA seal or a certifier's label.

For more information, visit the
National Organic Program (www.ams.usda.gov/nop).

The seal's scope and standards, however, are not fixed in stone. Since the release of these guidelines, players in the food industry have tried weakening them several times, including an attempt to remove the requirements for organic feed for organic-certified animals and to make acceptable previously prohibited antibiotics and pesticides.[17]

"Grassroots pressure has maintained strict standards each time," said Ronnie Cummins, founder of the Organic Consumers Association. "But there will always be petitions by industry to lower the standards and there will always be gray-area marketplace practices. We need to be constantly vigilant." For now, the USDA seal does offer certain guarantees about how the food we're eating was produced. (Some of the health benefits of these assurances are explored in the next chapter.)

WHAT THE ORGANIC SEAL DOES (AND DOESN'T) TELL US	
THE ORGANIC SEAL . . .	**BUT . . .**
gives you a solid assurance about how your food was grown. The certification includes strict requirements about farming practices (including what is allowed as fertilizer and pesticides), which is not true of nonorganic farming. The USDA seal also requires that certifiers visit farms to verify the reporting.	**doesn't mean food was grown without any pesticides.** Some naturally based pesticides as well as some synthetic pesticides deemed safe by the National Organic Standards Board are allowed. Allowable materials for use in organic production and processing are strictly regulated by the Board.
greatly reduces your exposure to synthetic chemicals. Because organic farming limits the use of synthetic chemicals, organic foods have been found to have significantly lower pesticide residues.	**doesn't guarantee you're exposed to *no* chemical residues.** Because some pesticides persist in our environment, some of these chemicals, including those long banned, appear as residues on *all* food, including organic.

THE ORGANIC SEAL . . .	BUT . . .
helps protect the environment. Organic farming practices can help protect the environment by limiting chemical use and encouraging composting, cover cropping, and other methods that improve soil quality.	**doesn't guarantee land stewardship.** The only way to be ensured of the quality of land stewardship is to know the farmer or company producing your food. The Cornucopia Institute has an online resource to find ratings of corporate ethics and farm production practices (cornucopia.org).
protects the health of farmers and farmworkers. Producers' exposure to toxic chemicals is dramatically reduced on organic farms.	**doesn't guarantee social justice.** The certification makes no stipulations about wages and other working conditions. The best guarantee of worker protection is a union label.
means that animals are raised more humanely than on industrial farms. The seal requires that animals have access to the outdoors, shade, shelter, fresh air, and direct sunlight. Growers must use organic feed and cannot use antibiotics or hormones in livestock production. (See page 86 for details.)	**doesn't *guarantee* that animals were raised humanely.** While the vast majority of organic farmers are ethical, a few companies are profiting from the organic seal but pursuing some pretty shady practices. Some have created massive industrial organic dairy farms, for instance, where animals technically have "access to" pasture but spend most of their time living in overcrowded, factory-farm conditions. Again, get to know who you are buying from and join with consumer advocacy groups to maintain the integrity of the organic seal.

THE ORGANIC SEAL . . .	BUT . . .
helps keep farmers on the land. Many small farmers have found that organic production enables them to be economically viable through price premiums and direct connections with their customers.	**doesn't tell us about the size (or type) of the farm or company.** Some organic farms and organic companies are part of the world's biggest food corporations. Others, like Organic Valley, are organized as cooperatives with family farms as active members. Look beyond the certification to know who you're buying from. (See page 64 for a breakdown of who owns what in the organic foods industry.)

Note: The provisions of the organic guidelines are subject to change. To find out the latest news and help maintain the integrity of the seal, visit us at eatgrub.org.

As some of the country's biggest food companies buy up smaller organic-certified businesses and launch their own organic lines, some small farmers who grow food using mostly organic practices are choosing *not* to be USDA-certified, stressing the importance of knowing their customers versus having a third-party seal. Interviews for this book with dozens of small-scale organic farmers in twelve states showed that more than half had chosen not to be USDA-certified. For some of these farmers, the several hundred dollars in costs and the administrative burden of certification is not worth it; having their customers know and trust them is enough.

Even those who had chosen to be certified organic underscored the importance of the connection between the grower and customer. Ed Lidzbarski, fifty-six, is one. A certified organic fruit and vegetable farmer, Lidzbarski has been farming in New Jersey for more than twenty-five years. "We're losing the trust of personal relationships," he said, "and replacing it with paper and signatures." Another farmer stressed that "certification shouldn't be a substitute for knowing and trusting your farmers and food sources." Of course, choosing to be certified and knowing your customers are not necessarily mutually exclusive! We can heed Lidzbarski's caution, seek out ways to get to know our farmers, and go beyond the seal.

Further learning: To learn more about organic foods read *The Organic Foods Sourcebook* by Elaine Marie Lipson. For more about the health and environmental consequences of eating sustainable and organic foods read *Genetically Engineered Food: A Self-Defense Guide for Consumers* by Ronnie Cummins and Ben Lilliston, *Seeds of Deception* by Jeffrey Smith, and *Omnivore's Dilemma* by Michael Pollen.

WHO ARE YOU BUYING YOUR ORGANICS FROM?

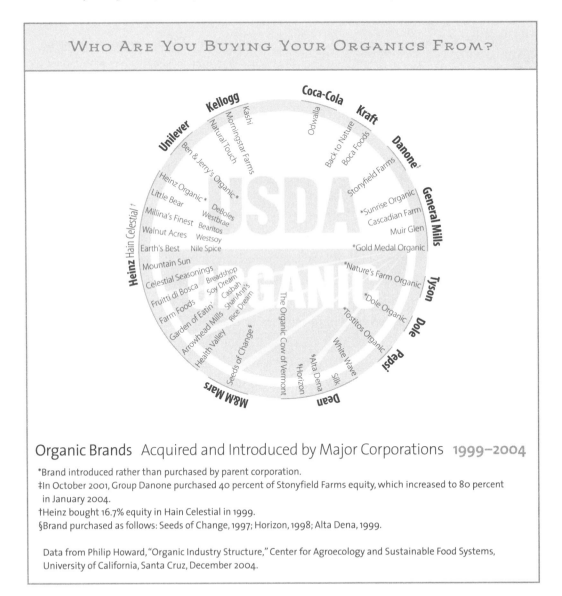

Organic Brands Acquired and Introduced by Major Corporations 1999–2004

*Brand introduced rather than purchased by parent corporation.

‡In October 2001, Group Danone purchased 40 percent of Stonyfield Farms equity, which increased to 80 percent in January 2004.

†Heinz bought 16.7% equity in Hain Celestial in 1999.

§Brand purchased as follows: Seeds of Change, 1997; Horizon, 1998; Alta Dena, 1999.

Data from Philip Howard, "Organic Industry Structure," Center for Agroecology and Sustainable Food Systems, University of California, Santa Cruz, December 2004.

Coda on Organics: Eat Whole Foods
(And We Don't Mean the Supermarket Chain)

In a world in which you can't escape branded, processed foods—even airplane aisles are now the domain of menus littered with TMs and ®s—it's no wonder that you now can find *processed* organic foods. While choosing organic can be a better choice, the healthiest choice is eating whole foods, as much as possible.

Whole foods are those that have gone through as little processing as possible to get from the ground, to your plate, and into your mouth. As one friend put it, you "eat the ingredients," not the final product. In whole foods, you also find the abundance of varieties in our food chain, explored in tasty depth in Bryant's recipes.

If you're choosing whole foods, you don't have to worry about whether you've deciphered the fine print of a food's packaging. Choosing whole foods is easy when you pick up a whole eggplant, apple, or bunch of spinach, but a little less obvious when you try to pick out whole grains. In the 2005 dietary guidelines the USDA underscored the importance of whole grains to our health, but that doesn't mean whole grains have become much easier to find.[18] "It's not as if you can go into the supermarket and ask for the whole-grain aisle!" says Michele Simon, founder of the Center for Informed Food Choices in Oakland, California.

Look for these varieties of whole grains, and choose organic when possible:

AMARANTH	BUCKWHEAT	MILLET	SPELT
BARLEY	KAMUT	OATS	WHOLE-GRAIN RYE
BROWN RICE	KASHA	QUINOA	WHOLE WHEAT

Along with the rich variety of these whole grains and vegetables and fruits, whole foods also include:

NUTS	SEEDS	BEANS AND LEGUMES
ALMONDS, WALNUTS	SUNFLOWER	LENTILS
HAZELNUTS, BRAZIL NUTS	FLAX	CHICKPEAS
CASHEWS	SESAME	KIDNEY BEANS

Further learning: A great sourcebook is *The New Whole Foods Encyclopedia* by Rebecca Wood.

Pillar 2: The Revival of the Local

At four in the morning on Terra Bella Farm in Hatton, Missouri, on any Saturday in September, you'll be awakened by the deafening roar of cicadas. Outside, the light from the barn will stream through the early-morning fog, illuminating a flatbed pickup piled eight feet high with organic produce. After strapping down the last boxes with frayed bungee cords, farmer DeLisa Lewis will head out east on Interstate 70 to a St. Louis farmers' market about 100 miles away.

On the way, Lewis will pass big box stores where the average food item will be jet-lagged and weary, having been bumped and bruised across thousands of miles before ending up in its customer's basket. In contrast, Lewis's offerings, like those of 19,000 other farmers who sell at weekly markets across the country, will have gone from field to truck to customer within just a few days (or less) of being picked. Lewis's customers know exactly how far their food has traveled; they can see it on her odometer.

I am drawn to Lewis's farm and this area to learn about how one region—the 85,000-person city of Columbia, Missouri, and its environs—is reviving a connection to the land and to local foods. Their efforts, a patchwork of brilliant ideas, are part of a global trend contributing to a quiet revolution in eating.

"When we said organic we meant local," said nutritionist and longtime organics advocate Joan Gussow the year the USDA standards were released. "We meant healthful. We meant being true to the ecologies of regions. We meant mutually respectful growers and eaters. We meant social justice and equality."[19]

The knitting together of community and food embodied in Lewis's work and that of dozens of others in the Columbia area are bringing to life Gussow's words.

Lewis and her partner, Holly Roberson, stumbled on the land that would become Terra Bella Farm in 1998. Roberson, who grew up in Columbia, wanted to farm close to home. Lewis, who had been farming in California for years, was up for the challenge of the Midwest weather.

So when the land went up for auction, Roberson, age twenty-five, and Lewis, thirty at the time, decided to make an offer on it. At the auction, the bidding came down to a battle between Roberson and Lewis and a man, they would later learn, who intended to turn the land into a hog factory farm operation.

When Lewis and Roberson outbid him and won the land, the crowd of locals—most decades older than them—burst into applause, shouting, "The girls got it! The girls got it!"

"Many people here still farm, and they wanted to see the land stay that way," Lewis said, by way of explanation. And it has.

Lewis and Roberson turned the 160 acres into a vibrant organic-certified farm, with 80 acres they rent out for grazing cattle, 40 acres for woods, and the rest for an orchard, vegetable and flower beds, a barn, and a farmhouse.

The farm's economic feasibility is tied completely to connections in their community: most of the farm's income comes from those weekly farmers' markets and the "shareholders" of their Community Supported Agriculture (CSA) program, community members who invest in the farm at the beginning of the year and receive weekly boxes of produce (and flowers, too) throughout the harvest season.

The local revival Lewis and Roberson are part of can be seen in the life choices of dozens of other area farmers, including Julie Walker and her husband, Tim.

The Walkers turned to farming in their forties, drawn to the idea of working for themselves and living closer to the land. They now farm forty minutes outside of Columbia on 144 acres, where they raise free-range chickens, turkeys, hogs, and cattle.

"It's hard work, but I love it," said Julie Walker who, with Tim, tends to 1,000 chickens, 150 turkeys, and dozens of hogs and cattle every year.

Like Terra Bella, the Walkers' farm is financially viable because they sell directly to their customers at farmers' markets and to local restaurants and grocery stores. (The Walkers also make it work because, like most of our nation's farmers, they also make off-farm income.)

"Eating local represents the best of the American spirit: sharing information and ideas and supporting each other," said Walker.

In town, various initiatives are helping consumers eat local, too, connecting them with newer farmers like the Walkers and farm families who have been on the land for generations.

At Walker Claridge's Root Cellar grocery store in Columbia almost every item in the bustling market is grown locally or made from local products. The day I visited, Claridge was busy in the store's attached kitchen, making value-added ketchup and pasta sauces from farm-fresh ingredients. Opened in 2001, the Root Cellar now offers products from more than 180 Missouri farmers, "90 percent of them from within one hundred miles," Claridge says.

Buying local foods not only strengthens community—as Julie Walker, DeLisa Lewis, and

Walker Claridge know firsthand—it strengthens local economies, too. "Local businesses spend more locally, unlike chain stores. They pay local managers, use local business services, advertise locally, and enjoy profits locally," says Michael Shuman, author of *Going Local* and an expert on building local economies.

"When we buy from local farmers, we know they're going to come back into town and spend it. The cycle keeps going," says Claridge. "So you can take the three hundred thousand in annual sales our store makes and multiply it by seven or more. That's our economic impact."

"Eating local is the most encouraging and significant change in the American diet today," says Brian Halweil, local-foods tracker and author of *Eat Here: Reclaiming Homegrown Pleasures in a Global Supermarket.* "It gives Americans a reason to be curious about how their food is raised, as opposed to the number of calories or grams of fat it has. That curiosity can shine a light on all those aspects of the American food system that have become problematic, whether it's animal rights, the environment, or abuse of farmworkers."

As Halweil observes, the eating-local trend is picking up around the country, flourishing with efforts like those in Columbia, where the city's population of 85,000 can now choose from two farmers' markets, two CSA farms, six farmstands, and dozens of area farms that offer naturally raised meat and dairy, fruits and vegetables, and flowers, berries, and honey, as well as nine grocery stores and twenty-nine restaurants that sell local foods.[20]

Around the country, the local food revival is also being encouraged by food policy councils, buy-local campaigns, and farm-to-college initiatives at schools and universities.

The University of Montana is one. Within a year of launching a buy-local campaign in 2004, the university was already purchasing nearly half a million dollars of local products. At Michigan State University, starting with a few identifiable local foods in 2004 the "Select Michigan" campaign saw a 10 to 27 percent increase in sales of local foods from participating stores.[21] The University of Iowa in Ames helped nearly double what restaurants, hospitals, retirement homes, colleges, and grocery stores in the region spent on local foods—from a quarter of a million to nearly half a million dollars in just one year.[22] "This is money that would have otherwise leaked out of our economy," said professor and campaign coordinator Kamyar Enshayan. (You'll read more about initiatives like these in "Chapter Seven: Out of the Kitchen, Into the Fire").

Of course, this trend is bumping up against the dominant one of processed and far-off food, epitomized by the box stores DeLisa Lewis passes every week. It's the trend seen in the farms that surround hers, stretching to the edge of the horizon. As far as the eye can see are monochromatic row crops—soy, corn, or sorghum—lined by small billboards that boast the pesticides at work. (Across from Terra Bella Farm one says "Pioneer: Results that Yield.") In comparison, Terra Bella looks chaotic: stalks of sunflowers just about to burst, zinnias buzzing with bees and butterflies. The land dips and curves; the rows bend around a field. Sweet pepper plants line beds newly planted with arugula next to rows still washed out from the recent rain.

When we buy food from farms like Terra Bella—when we choose Grub—we become part of this revival, too. We become part of the movement of people clapping right along with those old-timers at the farm auction, celebrating the vibrancy of Lewis's land in the face of the toxic uniformity of industrial agriculture.

Further learning: To explore the local food revival, check out Brian Halweil's *Eat Here,* Gary Nabhan's *Coming Home to Eat,* and Joan Gussow's *This Organic Life.*

PILLAR 3: THE JUST PLATE

One and a half hours south of San Francisco, right off Highway 1, a small sign propped against a funky wooden shop closed for the winter announces Swanton Berry Farm and its "California Certified Organic Farmer." Out across the highway, you can watch surfers with boards in the crooks of their arms jogging toward the Pacific and cars zooming south into Santa Cruz. At this time of year, Swanton Berry Farm may look unassuming, but it does what many say is impossible: the farm turns a profit while growing strawberries organically and employing unionized farmworkers.

This one farm, and others like it around the country, demonstrates that we can choose organic food and food grown by workers who are paid fair wages, treated with respect, and protected from workplace hazards, including pesticide exposure. (While I focus here on justice for farmworkers, the unfair treatment of workers in the food system extends from those who pick it to those who pack and process it to those who sell it to us.)

When Jim Cochran, now fifty-six, started Swanton Berry Farm with a business partner in 1983, they both were inspired by César Chávez and the United Farmworkers, the union Chávez cofounded in the 1960s to combat the brutal working conditions and poverty wages of California's farmworkers. From the beginning, Cochran also knew that he wanted to farm without chemicals—something many detractors said would be impossible to do with strawberries. As

I've mentioned, industrial strawberry farms apply heavy doses of the toxic fumigant methyl bromide, along with many other potentially toxic pesticides. In fact, more pesticides are used per acre on strawberries than any other crop in California.[23]

How has Cochran, then, successfully eschewed manmade chemicals? "Truth is, it's nothing earth shattering," said Cochran. "We just experimented. Starting without experience helped; we didn't have any preconceived ideas about how it all should work. We also knew a lot of old-timers who shared the tricks they used before chemicals, and we picked the brains of agricultural researchers at the university."

What began as a bold idea has grown into a sound business. Since 1987, Swanton Berry has been certified organic and now employs up to sixty people at the year's peak, all under a union contract.

"I was drawn to the union concept from the beginning," said Cochran. "In businesses without unions, it's very personal, which might sound good if the boss is great, but if he's not, you're in trouble. It's not so good to depend *only* on personal integrity. We have formalized, agreed-upon working conditions and the relationship with the union institutionalizes them: it's written into the contract."

Unionized workers are paid a fair wage, receive benefits (including family health insurance), and even collect pensions. As members of a union, workers are also protected from arbitrary discipline and harassment.

This seems like pretty basic stuff, right? And it should be. Only, it's the exception—not the rule—for the estimated 2.5 million farmworkers in the United States.[24] Making $8,000 on average annually, farmworkers toil under some of the most grueling conditions of any profession.[25] Farmworkers consistently rank in the top three most dangerous worker categories and are particularly vulnerable to workplace abuse because roughly half are undocumented immigrants.[26]

We often think of child labor as being a concern only for countries far away, but an estimated 300,000 to 800,000 farmworkers in the United States are under age eighteen,[27] and children as young as six have been found on our nation's farmland.[28] Working up to twelve-hour days for sometimes just two dollars a day, one in three child farmworkers suffers agriculture-related injuries.[29]

Farmworkers on industrial farms often come into close contact with toxic agricultural chemicals. Because farmworkers frequently bring their children into the fields, either to work, or because they don't have adequate childcare, farmworker children are also exposed to harmful pesticides.[30]

"Among just the illnesses reported, we've seen high levels of cancer, neurological damage, long-term memory loss, birth defects, and new data on potential learning disabilities among farmworker children," says Shelley Davis of the Farmworker Justice Fund.

In Florida, where commercial tomato growers use nearly 200 pounds of pesticides per acre compared with California's fifty, farmworkers have shown troubling health concerns.[31] In 2005, three children of migrant workers in Immokalee, Florida, were born with severe, and rare, birth defects.[32] But like many illnesses, both acute and mild, suffered by farmworkers exposed to a toxic mix of pesticides, identifying the offending chemical, and seeking retribution from the manufacturer, is exceedingly challenging. "The chances of being able to trace those birth defects to specific chemicals on the farm are slim," says Davis.

The EPA established the Worker Protection Standard in 1974 as its primary means of reducing the exposure of farmworkers to pesticides, but neither its protections nor its enforcement is adequate, say farmworker advocates. Many states perform worker safety inspections rarely, if at all. In 1998, five states reported that they had conducted none; in eleven states fewer than ten inspections had been conducted.[33] In California, which supposedly has some of the most rigorous protections, of the 4,069 reported pesticide violations in 2000, only 12 percent resulted in fines, and those fines averaged less than $400.[34]

"Farmworkers have been the human subjects—the *de facto* testers—of our farm chemicals," says Erik Nicholson, a farmworker advocate in the Pacific Northwest.

While growing foods organically means that workers are not exposed to potentially toxic farm chemicals, an organic seal doesn't necessarily promise us more than that. "A lot of people think that organic growers also treat their workers better, but some of them treat their workers just as badly as those farmers who use chemicals," says Marc Grossman, a longtime farmworker advocate with the United Farmworkers.

Is there a simple way to know "fair food" when you see it? We can look for union-made products, yes, but only a small percentage of farmworkers are unionized. We can also choose to buy from farmers we know and trust, but that is not an option for all of us or all of our food all the time.

So while we do have some options as consumers, supporting just food requires we do more than just shop right. We can also flex our citizen muscle, supporting union efforts and demanding more stringent enforcement of worker protection laws and other policies that help workers in the fields and factories.

The idea that we can help improve worker conditions may seem pie-in-the-sky, but we can be emboldened by recent examples of coalitions of farmworkers, citizens, students, and religious organizations that have changed company policy.

In 2005, the Florida-based Coalition of Immokalee Workers won a hard fought battle with Taco Bell and its parent company, Yum Brands. Since 2001, the workers and their allies around the country had been demanding better wages for the coalition's mostly immigrant farmworkers. The company finally agreed to the workers' demands, adding one penny per pound of tomatoes to their pay, increasing their wages by 80 percent.[35] This was a historic decision: never before had a fast-food giant caved to the demands of a worker right's organization.

"When we started this, it was like man going to the moon—nobody thought it was possible," said Lucas Benitez, of the Coalition of Immokalee Workers, to the Associated Press. "With the help of people around the country, we have built a way to go to the moon. Now we must continue moving forward."[36]

While we're working to create fair food in the United States, we do have a way to spot fair food imported from elsewhere: fair-trade certified products. The price of coffee or tea, like all commodities, is tied to the unpredictable fluctuations of the world market, with growers at the whim of speculation half a world away. Fair trade changes the dynamics of buying, selling, and trading. Guaranteeing a minimum "floor" price, often many times over the market price, fair-trade certified products provide farmers security and an essential source of income.

But fair trade is about more than just the money. Fair-trade farmers I've met from around the world have constantly underscored the other difference it makes in their lives. Without fair trade, their livelihood is at the mercy of those unpredictable world market prices and the middlemen they must sell to. They are kept in the dark about prices and how much traders are making off their products. With fair trade, farmers have full price disclosure; they operate as partners, not just input providers. They gain power. One fair-trade farmer from Nicaragua summed up the difference it has made to her and her community: "Fair trade," she said, "gives us back our dignity."

Since its founding in 1999, TransFair USA has certified products that have channeled more than $55 million in above-market pricing and additional income to more than 800,000 farmers and their families in 50 countries.[37] You can now find fair-trade coffee, tea, chocolate, bananas, mangoes, grapes, and more, in 35,000 stores around the country—even Dunkin' Donuts!

Further learning: For a historic perspective on working conditions in the U.S. food industry, read Upton Sinclair's *The Jungle.* For a more recent take, read Eric Schlosser's *Fast Food Nation* and *Reefer Madness.*

—◊—

In Italian, the words "knowledge" (*sapere*) and "taste" (*sapore*) differ by just one letter. Maybe this is no coincidence. Its relevance is certainly not lost on Carlo Petrini, founder of the Slow Food Movement, started in Italy in 1986. Petrini's movement, an "antidote to fast-food culture" as he says, has spawned tens of thousands of Slow Food members in 100 countries to work on ways to preserve traditional foods and promote environmental health and social equity through what we choose to eat.

Knowledge and taste are inextricably linked, Petrini stresses: knowledge changes taste. Knowing where your food comes from—the farmer who grew it, or the chemicals that were (or weren't) used to bring it to your plate—makes its flavors more delectable. Might we be able to taste fairness on our tongues? Petrini is reminding us of the connection between our minds, our hearts, and our taste buds. None of us, he says, merely consumes food; we are *coproducers.*

Our food choices build a market for certain foods, and not others. Our choices protect diversity and the health of our environment, or they help to destroy it. Our choices support certain norms of justice, or they undermine them.

Although fair food might just be the most challenging element of Grub to bring to life, justice on our plate may be one of the most important of all.

FIVE

Health 411

ORGANICS AND YOUR HEALTH

Tucked inside the glossy folder I received from the Fertilizer Institute—the trade association for (you guessed it!) the fertilizer industry—was a promotional DVD. In the video, a man with graying hair and smart-casual slacks stands in the middle of a field. He holds two identical-looking red apples. "Is this conventionally grown apple different nutritionally than this organically grown apple?" he asks.

"There have been numerous studies . . . to show that the nutritional value of these two apples is really the same. In fact, we can go to the literature and find 150 different studies [showing] these are really the same."[1] His name and title flash on the screen: Dr. Paul Fixen, Senior Vice President and Director of Research, Potash and Phosphate Institute.

Many of us reach for Grub—organic and locally grown food—because we believe it is nutritionally better for us, but is it? If you ask Fixen (or, it seems pretty much anyone else in the farm chemical industry), the answer is a resounding no.

"The fact is that conventionally grown food using these methods [chemical agriculture] is as safe and as nutritious as food that is produced by any other method," states CropLife America, the trade association for the developers, manufacturers, and distributors of pesticides, or as they call them "plant science solutions for agriculture and pest management."[2]

An American Chemical Society daylong symposium in 2004 asked, "Is organic food healthier than conventional food?" Funny, they arrived at the same answer: no.

Is this surprising? Industry execs have a big financial interest in our believing there's no difference between chemically treated and organic foods. And the media? They love controversy, and debunking popular ideas—such as organic foods are good for you—is a way to stir it up.

Front-page articles like one in Canada's largest circulation newspaper, the *Globe and Mail*, declared: "Organic Crops No More Nutritional."[3] The article cited an authoritative-sounding study, and featured an authoritative-looking graphic. But scratch the surface and you find holes in the evidence. Buried on page 7, the article mentions parenthetically that: "(The Guelph researchers who were contracted to do the work also stressed that the research was done with a very small sample and was not peer-reviewed.)"[4] Many readers wouldn't make it that far, appreciate the importance of the peer-review process, or know from the article that those conducting the study were based at Guelph University's Food Safety Network, which is funded in part by some of the world's biggest agrochemical companies, including DuPont Canada, Eli Lilly Canada Inc., Monsanto, and Syngenta.[5]

Despite what articles like this one might lead you to believe, evidence is starting to mount that organic foods may not only spare us from pesticide exposure—and in the case of meat and dairy, hormones and antibiotics—but offer us other health benefits as well.

Here's part of the answer. For decades now researchers have been investigating exactly what makes fruits and vegetables so darn good for us. The answer is, in part, plant metabolites called antioxidants, which foster plant health, and ours as well. There is general scientific consensus that antioxidants promote heart health, help prevent some cancers, slow the aging process, and decrease the risk of neurodegenerative diseases.[6]

In recent years, scientists interested in figuring out the potential nutritional benefits of organic fruits and vegetables have been devising ways to compare antioxidant levels across crops raised with chemicals and those without. The research is tricky to do. Antioxidant levels can vary for a whole range of different reasons; it's hard to pinpoint just what factors drive the variation.

But while more research is definitely needed, there are already some indications of the benefits of organic production. In 2003, *New York Times* journalist Marian Burros summarized: "Recent preliminary evidence suggests that the levels of certain nutrients, especially Vitamin C, some minerals and some . . . naturally occurring antioxidants . . . are higher in organically grown crops."[7]

Specific studies have found:

- organic marionberries, strawberries, and corn had between 30 and 50 percent more antioxidants than conventional ones;[8]
- juice extracted from organic vegetables had up to ten times the concentrations of flavonoids, which can act as powerful antioxidants;[9]
- organic crops surveyed in a Danish study had between 10 and 50 percent higher antioxidant levels than chemically grown crops.[10]

In a state of the science review, the Organic Center for Education and Promotion in the United States found that of the fifteen studies with quantitative evaluations of organically grown versus chemically grown crops, thirteen of them found higher antioxidant levels in the organically grown varieties, on average 30 percent higher.[11]

Why might organic foods exhibit greater levels of antioxidants? Organic practices create healthier plants because—this may seem paradoxical at first—they're forced to defend themselves against disease and insects. Under such stress, plants produce defense compounds, which in turn create the good-for-us antioxidants, and can produce higher-quality foods.[12] These same defense compounds are often health-promoting, like resveratrol, found in red grapes, which has many health benefits, including lowering bad cholesterol.[13]

The soil on organic fields is also different. Organic farming feeds the soil, supplying it with carbon, which supports a whole underground, and out-of-sight, ecosystem. A gram of soil can contain ten thousand species of microbes, microbes which, in turn, feed the plant. "This is how plants evolved," says agroecologist Don Lotter. "When industrial farms fertilize the plant directly, they short circuit the whole process."

But the science evaluating overall nutritional benefits of eating an organic diet compared with a diet from chemical farms is "still in its infancy," says Bob Scowcroft of the Organic Farming Research Foundation. To really compare organic and conventional diets, we'll need long-term studies that look beyond specific nutritional differences. In the meantime, we can be encouraged by the preliminary research that choosing organic might not only be more pleasing to our taste buds, but kinder to our health, too.

SUPERHERO PRODUCE: THE NUTRITIONAL PUNCH OF LOCAL

"Perhaps the greatest culprit behind lost nutritional value is simply that old nemesis, the passage of time," weighs in central Illinois organic farmer Henry Brockman, forty-one, about the health benefits of organic and local foods. Brockman should know. Every week he delivers selections from 450 varieties of dozens of different fruits and vegetables to a farmers' market near Chicago, where customers have been known to arrive as early as six in the morning—flashlights in hand—to get the crème-de-la-freshly-picked-crème.

"As soon as a vegetable is picked it begins losing nutritional value," says Brockman.[14] The bruising and battering of travel can cause oxidation and loss of nutrients. One study found that just three days after having been harvested, green beans had lost 60 percent of their vitamin C, and leeks had lost more than 50 percent of their total carotene, notes Brockman.[15] In other words, eating fresh (not just organic) is good for your health, too.

Says Brockman, "I won't argue that the organic produce sitting in Fresh Fields, Jewel, or Kroger is more nutritious than its conventional cousin. But I will argue fiercely that my small-scale, locally grown, locally sold organic produce raised on rich and healthy soil under natural conditions is."[16]

These benefits of eating fresh, local foods may confirm what many of us have long sensed instinctively: much is better for you in that crunchy, bursting-with-flavor Fuji from Hepworth Farms a few hours outside of New York City than in that apple from New Zealand carried along conveyor belts, in the bellies of jet planes and innards of trucks; sprayed with chemicals and watching the clock on the shelves of a distribution plant; then sent out again, across roads and more roads, and resting for days in a grocery display before making its way finally to your grocery cart, and finally, finally to your mouth.

WHOLE FOODS AND YOUR HEALTH

Whether we're choosing organic foods or not, we can also heed Jack LaLanne's lifelong mantra: "If man made it, don't eat it!" The 1950s fitness guru and nutrition pioneer got it right long ago and his spunk—and two hours of exercise a day at age ninety—seem to prove it. Whether we choose organic or not the best choice for our bodies is whole food. Unfortunately, in our packaged, branded, fast-food culture we've come a long way from his most basic and healthy precept.

"I don't think the average American realizes how truly bad our food is by the time we eat it, how much of the good stuff is gone, how many valueless calories come in," says Dr. Charles Benbrook, Chief Scientist of the Organic Center for Education and Promotion.

Unprocessed, whole foods are naturally higher in fiber and lower in fat, sodium, sugar, and additives than processed foods. Whole grains, which just got a big thumbs-up in the new USDA dietary guidelines, are a far nutritional cry from the processed grains that make up most of the chips and bread, pasta and baked goods we find on grocery shelves and in fast-food outlets.

Processed grains were originally developed not for our health, but for aesthetics, practicality . . . and profit. By extracting the outside (the bran), food companies could achieve the white, fluffy quality that became symbolic of good taste, first embodied in the now infamous Wonder Bread. With the delicate center (the germ) extracted, products could also last longer on the shelf.

Only one small problem: the bran and the germ are the most nutritious parts of the plant. Bran is a natural fiber, abundant with minerals and proteins. Fiber also helps regulate blood sugar by slowing down the conversion of starches to glucose so that the speed and intensity with which the glucose hits your bloodstream—what's called the "glycemic load"—is lessened. The germ is the plant's "embryo," storing nutrients—proteins, minerals, and vitamins.

With the bran and germ gone, what's left—the endosperm—is basically just starch. It's "the cheapest and most abundant part," says Mollie Katzen, who has been spreading the whole foods gospel, with cookbooks like *The Enchanted Broccoli Forest*, since 1974.

So much of what's good for us goes missing when whole grains get refined and processed that the feds even passed recommendations for spiking grain products with some of the lost essential nutrients. (We sometimes fortify foods to address public health crises, too. For example, folate has been added to grain products since 1998 in an effort to reduce birth defects.)

But nature knows best. New science continually humbles us, revealing that we're only beginning to understand the complexity of foods and their benefits to us in their whole state. An explosion of research in the past decade has provided new evidence, for example, of phytochemicals we didn't even know existed, and has delivered new understanding of the synergy of nutrients and micronutrients in whole foods. So even though some processed foods have been enriched with vital nutrients we know get lost in the processing, we miss out, big time, on the full health benefits of whole foods.

Listen to LaLanne: it's best we get our nutrients from their unadulterated source by eating a varied diet of whole grains and fruits and vegetables. And by "fruits and vegetables" we mean the real deal—not high-fructose corn syrup and water disguised as fruit juice, sodium-saturated canned veggies, or so-called fruit snacks with no remnants of fruit in them at all!

Researchers have been exploring the health benefits of a diet rich in fruits and veggies for a long time now and the verdict is certainly in. We also know whether organic or not, few of us are meeting our dietary needs of whole foods. Scientists at Tufts University estimate that the average American consumes "less than a third of the dietary antioxidants needed to take full advantage of [their] health-promoting benefits."[17] Dr. Walter Willett and colleagues at the Harvard School of Public Health spell out some of the benefits.

WHY YOU'LL BE GLAD YOU EAT YOUR FRUITS AND VEGGIES

- **Cancer:** Fruit and vegetable consumption can lower risk of a variety of cancers, including those of the mouth, kidneys, lungs, and ovaries.
- **Heart disease and stroke:** Eating fruits and vegetables can lower your chances of developing heart disease and stroke by as much as 30 percent.
- **High blood pressure:** Eating a diet full of fruits, vegetables, and low-fat dairy products (and limited consumption of saturated and total fat) can reduce blood pressure.
- **High cholesterol:** A fruit- and vegetable-rich diet has been shown to decrease cholesterol levels.
- **Vision:** Fruits and vegetables help keep your eyes healthy and your vision strong.

Adapted from Eat, Drink, and Be Healthy.

Further learning: If you'd like to delve more deeply into the health benefits of whole foods, read *Eat, Drink, and Be Healthy: The Harvard Medical School Guide to Healthy Eating,* by Walter Willett, MD, codeveloped with the Harvard School of Public Health.

ATTACK OF THE KILLER LETTUCE AND APPLE JUICE ASSASSINS

Maybe, to you, the health benefit of a Grub diet—locally grown, organic, whole foods—is a no-brainer. But as the demand for this kind of food has increased, so has the venom of its handful of detractors trying to get us to question our common sense. (You'll see it doesn't take a large cast of characters to cast doubt, however unfounded, on a critical public issue. It just takes a well-funded one.)

Among the most vocal is Dennis Avery, who made a big splash on *20/20* several years ago when he used the national platform to warn that organic produce is likely to be infested with "nasty strains of bacteria."[18] Why? Because it is "fertilized with manure," was Avery's short answer.[19] A wide-eyed Barbara Walters closed the segment by asking, "I've been buying organic food. It is more expensive. But it isn't dangerous?"[20]

Avery certainly went for the "ew-gross" response by linking organic farming to manure. Yes, organic farmers can use manure for fertilizer, but only under strict guidelines: an organic farmer must wait 120 days after applying manure before harvesting or ninety days for food, like oranges, that doesn't come into direct contact with the soil. Within thirty to sixty days, the *E. coli* pathogen of particular concern is naturally eliminated from manure.[21]

"The number one thing to remember is that manure is used in conventional agriculture, too, but no one regulates it," says organic farmer Rose Koenig, a member of the National Organic Standards Board. Industrial farms are also free to use municipal sewage sludge as fertilizer and, for feed, slaughterhouse waste, which can include bonemeal, blood, and even chicken feces. Talk about gross!

Avery's campaign against organic food began long before that *20/20* appearance. Two years earlier, in 1998, Avery alleged that "According to recent data compiled by the U.S. Centers for Disease Control, people who eat organic and 'natural' foods are eight times as likely as the rest of the population to be attacked by a deadly new strain of *E. coli* bacteria (O157:H7)."[22]

Scary stuff, right?

Don't worry; the evidence tells a different story. You can find the contradicting data online. Anyone can, including the journalists who have repeated Avery's claims without doing even the most basic armchair sleuthing. You can also read online official retractions to some of Avery's assertions by *20/20* host John Stossel, as well as a refutation from the Centers for Disease Control.[23]

Avery bases his allegation on CDC figures from 1996, which he says attributed roughly 500 illnesses that year to the deadly form of *E. coli,* one-quarter of them from natural or organic foods. These cases came from two "outbreak clusters": one, from organically grown lettuce, the other from "natural" apple juice.[24]

Avery's implication is that the lettuce in question was contaminated by manure in organic agriculture. In fact, it was manure of *non*organic cattle in a packing facility abutting the field that contaminated the lettuce.[25] And the apple juice? It was natural, yes, but it was also unpasteurized, which resulted in the *E. coli* contamination, the only such outbreak in the company's history. The company, Odwalla, now owned by Coca-Cola, immediately launched a product recall and changed their production process to prevent a recurrence.[26]

I was on the debate team in high school. If I had tried to build a case against organics the way Avery does—using data that doesn't support my thesis, sources that contradict my conclusions, a biased sample year and small sample size—I would have been laughed off the team. But Avery's scare-mongering campaign is still making the rounds years later.

If you ever wondered how urban legends stick, consider the following: in 2004, a full *six* years after Avery's original allegation, a Lexis-Nexis search revealed an article halfway around the world, claiming: "In the U.S. the rate of recall of organic foods is running at eight times the rate of recall of regular products."[27]

When I inquired via e-mail, the author, Owen McShane of the New Zealand–based Center for Resource Management, confirmed that Avery was the source for his allegation.[28] In 1998, Avery had (falsely) claimed that people who eat organic or "natural" foods are "eight times as likely" to be afflicted by *E. coli* O157:H7. Here, years—and several twists—later, organic foods are deemed eight times as likely to be recalled.

WILL THE REAL SOURCE OF FOODBORNE HEALTH THREATS PLEASE STAND UP?

While the jury may still be out on the exact nutrient-by-nutrient benefits of eating organic, the jury is certainly back—and has rendered its verdict—about what you *don't* get when you eat organic foods. Exactly what Avery's fear-mongering distracts us from. The cases Avery highlighted, for instance, made up less than 1 percent of the total 22,607 cases of foodborne illnesses in his year of choice.[29] In other words, he ignored over *99 percent* of illnesses from *E. coli* and *Salmonella* and other foodborne illnesses associated with industrial farming.

The Centers for Disease Control estimate that 76 million people—or roughly one out of four of us—suffer from foodborne illnesses each year in the United States, accounting for 325,000 hospitalizations and more than 5,000 deaths.[30] These illnesses cost us between $5 and $6 billion a year in direct medical expenses and lost productivity annually, according to the National Institutes of Health.[31] *E. coli* O157:H7 alone accounts for roughly 73,000 illnesses every year, with thousands of hospitalizations and dozens of deaths from infection and complications.[32] None of these illnesses has come from organic food.

Ironically (and tragically), the real culprit is not organic farming, but the very industrial farming Avery advocates. The virulent *E. coli* strain O157:H7 wasn't first reported until 1982.[33] It emerged as a direct result of the introduction of factory farming and the conditions it breeds: close confinement of animals, increased antibiotic use, and poor hygiene in the slaughter, production, and distribution of meat.[34] Weak standards and lax enforcement in meat processing plants has also allowed this strain of *E. coli* and other increasingly potent foodborne pathogens to spread. Journalist Christopher D. Cook notes that two-thirds of U.S. meat inspectors surveyed in September 2000 agreed that under current federal regulations, "there have been instances when they have not taken direct action against contamination (feces, vomit, metal shards, etc.) that they observed."[35]

Foodborne illnesses in general persist in large part because of the promotion of industrial farming and the failure of policy to protect our public health, not because of the spread of organic farming. A foray into the federal food recalls website might help you capture the scope of the problem: in just one year, 2002, ConAgra recalled 19 million pounds of potentially *E. coli*–tainted beef, enough for one-fourth of the entire U.S. population to have eaten a burger contaminated with the deadly strain of the bacteria.[36] That same year, poultry processor Pilgrim's Pride recalled 27.4 million pounds of meat—or 146 million servings.[37]

In 2004, 2.3 million pounds of meat was recalled by the USDA, the majority from concerns about *Listeria* and *E. coli* contamination, but also included such unwelcome surprises as chicken "adulterated with extraneous materials (small pieces of metal)" and meat containing shards of glass and fragments from a handheld calculator.[38] Yikes. Organic and "natural" foods did not account for even one recall.

Something to keep in mind when you learn about these federal recalls: the Food and Drug Administration does not have the power to protect our health by ordering mandatory recalls. These recalls are *voluntary*. Industry decides, and thousands of consumers are sickened, and some die, because of it.

OUR CHEMICALS, OURSELVES

Yes, contamination by pathogens brings acute illness, even death, but the threat of chemical residues and exposure may be just as serious, only harder to detect. Low-level exposure to toxins in our food can cause illnesses afflicting us years, sometimes even decades, after initial exposure.

Organic detractors, however, pooh-pooh the chemical threat. "What is the health trade-off for this abundance, produced with the help of chemicals? None," says Avery.[39] Referring to Rachel Carson's predictions in *Silent Spring*, Avery says, "We . . . know now that Ms. Carson's fears of widespread human cancer from pesticides have not borne out."[40]

"A little bit of poison or pollution can do you good . . ." contends another chemical agriculture proponent, former British minister of Parliament Lord Dick Taverne and author of *The March of Unreason*.

How I wish they were right. We'd have a lot less to worry about. But the facts prove these assertions, in a word, wrong.

In the past twenty years, the incidence of childhood cancers has been steadily increasing. Cancer is now the second leading cause of death among children under age fourteen.[41] Among adults, brain tumors, lymphoma, breast, prostate, and testicular cancer have all increased over the past few decades. Many of the cancers on the rise are those whose appearance has been tied to pesticide exposure, including the farm chemicals found as residues on our food and in our groundwater.[42]

And what about farmers? Citing what sounds like credible research, Taverne says: "More than 30 separate investigations of about 500,000 people have shown that farmers, millers, pesticide-users, and foresters, occupationally exposed to much higher levels of pesticide than the general public, have much lower rates of cancer overall."[43]

I checked his source and it was 300,000, not 500,000 people, but never mind the small stuff . . . the point is Taverne is right, sort of. Farmers *do* have significantly less cancer overall than the general public, mainly because of a healthier lifestyle. "They tend to smoke less, exercise more, but they have substantially more cancers of particular varieties," says Dr. Michael Alavanja, with the Agricultural Health Study. "This we suspect is due to occupational exposure."[44] Dr. Alavanja should know. His multi-year study is monitoring the health of nearly 90,000 farmers, farm families, and pesticide applicators in the United States, investigating the links between pesticide exposure and a range of serious diseases.

So Taverne gets it half right; too bad the other half of the story contradicts the first.

Avery likes to say that manmade chemicals are "no more dangerous than natural chemicals."[45] Try telling that to the farmers.

Tell it to Cheryl and Mike Rogowski, brother-and-sister farmers who lost two uncles, farmers in their early fifties, to kidney disease. Or to farmer John Kinsman, who was hospitalized from agricultural chemical exposure before he turned to organic farming. Or to any of the other farmers I've met from the rolling hills of southeastern Poland to Wisconsin dairyland, from the foothills of the Indian Himalayas to black-dirt country of New York, who *all* have experienced death or too-close-for-comfort illness from exposure to toxic farm chemicals.

Try telling Guy Jones. "I knew I was getting sicker and sicker, but none of my doctors could tell me what was wrong," said Guy Jones, a farmer in Blooming Hill, New York.

"I finally saw a doctor who took one look at my tests and asked if I'd ever worked on a farm. That's when I knew I had gotten sick from the spraying," Jones said. "Not because I was being stupid, but because I was overexposed to parathion and malathion—pesticides everybody was working with."

"I hated spraying anyhow," Jones added. "No farmer wakes up in the morning and says, 'Ooh, great, I get to spray today.' They're just trying to make a living. They have to have perfect-looking products and they're only growing one crop—so they have to spray."

And it's this spraying, as I've discussed, which leaves chemical residues on the food we eat.

In one review of more than 94,000 food samples, at least one pesticide residue was detected on nearly *three-quarters* of all chemically grown food.[46] Only one-quarter of organic samples had residues, and at much lower levels. Most of the pesticide residues found on organic foods were those from chemicals long been banned here—such as DDT, dieldrin, and chlordane—but still found in the environment, and as these tests show, in our food supply. These residues find their way not only into our environment and our food, but into our bodies, too.[47]

Eating organic foods is one way to lower your risk of exposure. "Pesticides may . . . contribute the largest proportion of dietary risk, simply because so many different residues from pesticides classified as possible or probable carcinogens are permitted on a large number of foods," writes Yale University's John Wargo in *Our Children's Toxic Legacy.*[48]

It is a choice that is particularly important for children. Comparing preschoolers who ate mostly organic and those who consumed mostly conventional foods, researchers found that in the children who didn't eat an organic diet organophosphate pesticide residues were six times higher. (Organophosphates are among the most acutely toxic pesticides: they interfere with the nervous system and can cause developmental or reproductive harm and some cancers. Some can also be endocrine disrupters.) As one of the study's authors pointed out: "Organic produce appears to provide a relatively simple way for parents to reduce their children's exposure to pesticides."[49]

Eating local foods is another way to decrease our exposure to pesticide residues. Some of the most toxic pesticides are banned in the United States but still produced here and shipped overseas. U.S. customs records from 1996, for instance, showed that on average one ton a day of DDT, banned in the United States in 1972, was still being shipped from our nation's ports.[50] Between 1997 and 2000, the United States exported 3.2 billion pounds of pesticides, many considered "extremely hazardous" by the World Health Organization and 65 million pounds of which were pesticides that had been either "forbidden" or "severely restricted" here.[51] When we import food back into the country and then consume it, we're completing what has been called the "circle of poison."[52]

Eating low on the food chain is another way to improve the safety of your diet: nonorganic meat has been shown to have higher concentrations of agricultural chemical residues. It makes sense. Factory-farmed meat is raised on pesticide-treated feed, pesticides that can become concentrated in animal fat.[53] As you'll see in the next chart, factory-farmed animals are also raised on such tasty treats as animal by-products (including blood and bonemeal), growth hormones such as rBGH used in dairy cows, antibiotics, arsenic-based drugs, sewage sludge, and more.

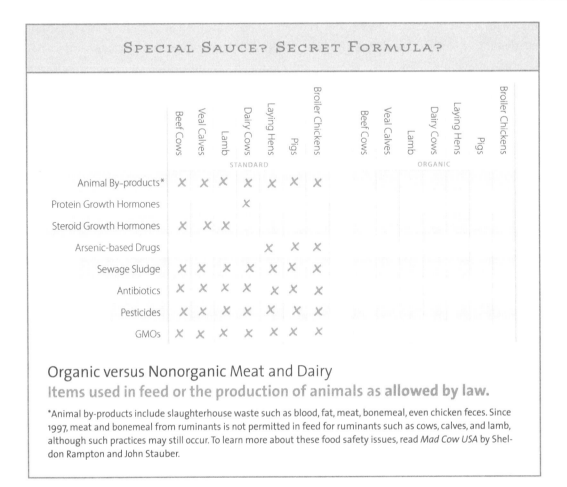

	Beef Cows	Veal Calves	Lamb	Dairy Cows	Laying Hens	Pigs	Broiler Chickens	Beef Cows	Veal Calves	Lamb	Dairy Cows	Laying Hens	Pigs	Broiler Chickens
	STANDARD							ORGANIC						
Animal By-products*	X	X	X	X	X	X	X							
Protein Growth Hormones					X									
Steroid Growth Hormones	X	X	X											
Arsenic-based Drugs					X	X	X							
Sewage Sludge	X	X	X	X	X	X	X							
Antibiotics	X	X	X	X	X	X	X							
Pesticides	X	X	X	X	X	X	X							
GMOs	X	X	X	X	X	X	X							

Organic versus Nonorganic Meat and Dairy
Items used in feed or the production of animals as allowed by law.

*Animal by-products include slaughterhouse waste such as blood, fat, meat, bonemeal, even chicken feces. Since 1997, meat and bonemeal from ruminants is not permitted in feed for ruminants such as cows, calves, and lamb, although such practices may still occur. To learn more about these food safety issues, read *Mad Cow USA* by Sheldon Rampton and John Stauber.

A MANIFESTO OF INTERDEPENDENCE

Chemical industry execs will persist with assertions about what is safe and clean; public-interest advocates will persist with research to protect our health from unnecessary toxins. As agribusiness feels even more threatened by those who've ordered the wake-up call, these food debates—about organic foods' benefits, about the nutritional bang from local and whole foods, about the real food threats—will undoubtedly heat up. The agrichemical industry is surely aware that the market for organic, local foods is growing, that citizens are intensifying pressure on our policymakers for stricter pesticide and animal treatment standards.

As these sides continue to battle it out, it is critical that we dig for the facts ourselves and use our common sense, constantly asking questions and expecting the truth—not PR fluff.

Foodborne illnesses and the toxic exposure to chemical residues in our food are frightening, yes. These exposures are also avoidable—to a certain extent, at least. While we're pushing for stricter standards, greater government oversight, and corporate responsibility, we can choose whole foods, fresh foods, and meat and dairy (if we choose to consume them) from farmers and distributors we know and trust.

When we make these choices, we're not only making a choice for our individual health, we're helping change a whole way of farming that will have ripple effects far beyond us.

Pesticides, as I've discussed, pollute our soil, waterways, and air, causing untold numbers of illnesses (and sometimes even death) among farmworkers and farmers. Every time we demand food grown without chemicals and genetically modified organisms, when we love our produce's blemishes, we're helping farmers jump off the industrial farm treadmill and land on their feet.

Choosing Grub, we are saving lives.

When scientists documented the health hazards of cigarettes, we as a nation shifted the way we thought about smoking and supported policy-making that reflected this reframing. In the past thirty years, as norms have changed, we've seen bans on smoking in restaurants, bars, and public places, as well as tobacco lawsuits with multimillion dollar settlements.

Less than thirty years ago, hospitals carried cigarette vending machines in their hallways. Doctors (and nurses) would consult with their patients as smoke swirled around them, and overfull ashtrays sat on their desks. My uncle, a cardiologist, told me he made a stink about the cigarette vending machines at his hospital nearly thirty years ago. The higher-ups thought he was being ridiculous. Cigarette vending machines in hospital waiting rooms? Today it seems inconceivable.

Smoking is no longer considered (just) an individual health problem; it is a public health issue. We can help bring about a similar conceptual shift about the practices used to produce our nation's food supply. We can wake up to realize and reject the wastefulness and cruelty of factory-farmed meat, the real inefficiency of our industrial farms. In an increasingly interconnected world, where a chemical sprayed, or genetically modified crop planted, in California (or Chile or China) will wend its way throughout the environment, our individual choice for Grub takes on a whole new meaning.

We don't need to buy it, literally.

It's time we turn the "you are what you eat" truism on its head: I am, in effect, what you eat; you are what I eat. It's time to awaken to a diet of interdependence.

Interlude:
Cheat Sheet for
the Cocktail Party

I was at a dinner party the other night and got to talking about my work. "It's a rip-off," one of the guests said, when I mentioned organic foods. "It's a big propaganda campaign to get us to pay more for our food, and what difference does it make anyway?"

Maybe you've had a conversation like this one and wished you could instantly conjure up the most compelling reasons for Grub. Well, here's a cheat sheet to help; consider it Grub Cliff's Notes. It might help next time you're in the hot seat. When you are, though, there's no need to jump from the hot seat to a pedestal. It's safe to assume that most of us share common values: that we like clean air and clean water, that we'd like to see people in the world fed and healthy and treated fairly, that we would like for ourselves and our loved ones to live long lives, free from cancer, debilitating obesity, and other serious illnesses. So start from there—after all, that's what Grub is all about.

Top Ten Reasons Why Eating Grub Is a Very Good Idea

10. No More Mouthfuls of Additives

Processed foods contain all kinds of additives—from sweeteners and colorings to preservatives—many of which have been linked to illnesses, including allergies, headaches, asthma, growth retardation, and heart disease.

9. Worry Less about Consuming Food that May Make You Sick

While scientists study which pesticides on the market are carcinogenic or are endocrine-disrupters and while regulators battle it out with the food industry, we can ensure peace of mind by choosing food grown without chemicals and organic meat and dairy.

8. Opt Out of Being a Guinea Pig for Genetically Modified Foods

While we're doing the research to understand how GMOs affect our environment (and our bodies), you don't have to be the guinea pig. Since labeling GMOs in food is not required in the United States (as of this writing), choosing organic or "Non-GMO" or "GMO-free" is the only way to ensure you are not eating GMOs.

7. Miss Out on Hydraulic Fluid in Your Burger

With strict guidelines for acceptable feed, organic, sustainably raised meat lessens your risk of exposure to foodborne pathogens and other contaminants (even hydraulic fluid, calculator parts, metal shards—you get the idea). Eating organic meat and dairy also means you're not consuming products raised with hormones and antibiotics.

6. Get a Nutritional Bang for Your Hard-Earned Buck

Whole foods have been shown to have higher nutritional content and more fiber than their processed foods counterparts. Evidence for the nutritional benefits of organic food is also mounting.

5. Claim Your Power

You decide exactly what's in your food; you control the salt, sugar, and fat. The more you prepare meals for yourself the more you know how much of that stuff is in there.

4. Celebrate the Spirit of Your 'Hood

When you eat local foods, you're supporting local businesses and farmers. The local economy will thank you for it.

3. Earn Karma Points

When you raise your fork, or slurp from your spoon, you know there's a better chance that no farmworkers, farmers, or processing workers were exploited in the process of getting the food to you.

2. Protect Food and Cultural Diversity and Food Traditions

Farmers throughout history have saved and shared seeds and raised a diverse variety of plants and animals. When we choose Grub, we help keep these traditions alive.

1. "Yum"—Enough Said

This could well be the number one reason for many of us; let's face it, this food also tastes better—way better.

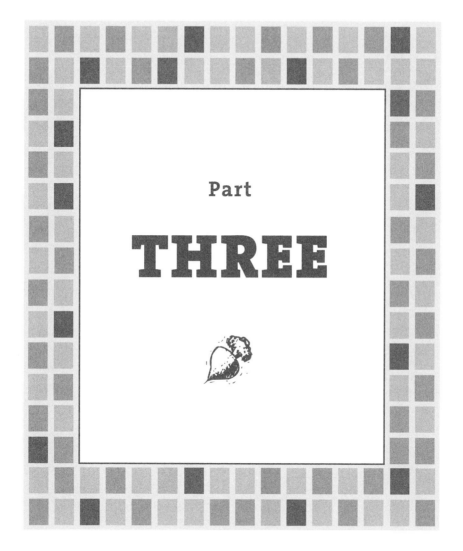

Part

THREE

SIX

Seven Steps to a Grub Kitchen

I feel slightly disingenuous writing this today of all days. From my desk I can see my kitchen and in my kitchen I can see it's been a while since I got to the farmers' market, even longer since my last trip to the grocery store. Okay, so today my kitchen may not be the paragon of Grub-ness. But here is where the "slightly" of "slightly disingenuous" comes in: shifting our diet in a healthier direction doesn't mean we get it right 100 percent of the time. The key is to create habits—habits of mind and habits of shopping—that make it easier for us to have good days and harder to have bad ones.

Welcome to the nitty-gritty: seven steps to help you get into the Grub habit and create for yourself a user-friendly kitchen. Consider these steps just friendly suggestions, not a dogmatic tract. You're the one cooking in your kitchen, after all, and thankfully we're each unique. Our kitchens should be, too. Most important, eating and cooking this way should be fun, and done right, it will be.

These steps may seem simple to some of you, to some they may feel daunting. Either way, having a partner in crime (or two, or three) as you go through these steps can make the process more enjoyable. Compare notes, swap ideas, share tips. By the time you get to step seven-and-a-half, you'll really have something to celebrate—together.

Step 1: Get Off the Bus

Several years ago, on the 'round-the-world journey for my first book, *Hope's Edge,* I found myself on the edge of Nairobi in an airy guesthouse surrounded by towering jacaranda trees. I was interviewing Professor Wangari Maathai who, at the time, was struggling to keep afloat her Green Belt Movement, a grassroots, women-led effort she launched in the 1970s to avert desertification in her home country of Kenya.

Challenging the corruption and environmental abuse of President Moi's regime, the movement had faced serious roadblocks for years. Maathai and members of the movement had even been beaten and jailed by the government for their work. When we met, she was unsure whether the movement would have the funds to continue. (No one then could have predicted that four years later she would be awarded the Nobel Peace Prize.)

That day, Maathai shared one of the ways she helped women claim their power to make a difference: a workshop she called "The Wrong Bus Syndrome."

"We all know how much trouble we would be in if we got on the wrong bus, headed in the wrong direction," she would say to the group of women gathered for the workshop. "But if you are on a bus and discover it's headed in the wrong direction, what would you do?"

"Well, of course you'd get off the bus," the women would answer.

So what could possibly make anyone stay on the wrong bus? "You'd been given the wrong information, you didn't know you were on the wrong bus." "You didn't have enough money to get on another bus." "You didn't know there was another bus," would be some of the common responses. Maathai would then lead the women through a discussion of their lives, their hardships, the policies of the president's regime.

"It is much like being on the wrong bus," she would suggest. "We as a nation are headed in the wrong direction, and each of us has the ability to make the conscious choice to get off." Encapsulating this message, the movement's slogan is, simply, "As for me, I've made a choice."

If you've read this far maybe you, too, would agree we're generally making the wrong choices—that is, on the wrong bus—when it comes to our food and farming. You wouldn't be alone. So the question is why aren't *more* of us getting off the bus? Part of the answer, as I've said, is that many of us don't have the information to know we're on the wrong bus. (Hopefully, this book has already helped remedy that!) But one of the other reasons is that many of us feel it's too hard to get off: It's too expensive, some protest. It takes too much time, others say. So first let's tackle these two concerns that stop many of us from getting off the bus to begin with.

Getting Off the Bus: Time

More and more of us are working more hours, for more days a year, for more years of our life. We work on average 350 hours longer every year than our European counterparts, nearly *nine full weeks.* We are—my time-strapped friends—the only industrialized country with no mandatory paid vacation.[1]

Yes, it's true, we have less time than we used to, and many feel that choosing Grub will suck up what little of it we have left. But maybe we can find more time in our lives than we thought we had. Try your own time audit: are there patterns you can change to incorporate these principles of eating into your life? After all, somehow the average one of us is finding four hours every day to watch television.

You may be surprised to discover that following these principles won't necessarily take more of your time. You can cook many simple, whole foods meals in the time it would take to prepare a packaged meal, and in often less time than it would take for you to go out for a meal, even at a so-called fast-food restaurant.

You may also discover that as you integrate these habits into your life, your relationship with time and food shifts. You might actually (gasp!) find that suddenly the time spent cooking gives you peace of mind, that meals provide new connections to your family and friends, to your own health. You may find yourself, with your new habits, not worried about the time and Grub, at all.

Getting Off the Bus: Money

I was thinking about the cost of eating organic and healthy the other day when I found myself, hungry, on Manhattan's tony Upper East Side. I had just attended a black-tie awards dinner in honor of Wangari Maathai, but the closest I had come to the entrée was when a waiter dropped a filet mignon on my jacket. So before heading home, I decided to pick up something at a nearby supermarket.

As the cashier rang up my purchases, I looked up just in time to see "Organic Nectarines $2.86" flash on the register—for two nectarines slightly bigger than golf balls. I asked the cashier to put them aside. A few items later, she punched in two organic grapefruits at $5.94. I didn't buy those, either. When she got to the organic cashews, she held up the small container and said: "Seven ninety-nine," adding, "they're *organic*." We put those aside, too.

In this Food Emporium in the shadow of the Queensboro Bridge, organics were more expensive—big time. If you do the math, those unpurchased items add up to more than three hours of work at minimum wage (probably what that checkout worker gets paid).

But eating organic foods and a healthy, whole-foods diet doesn't have to make such a dent in our wallet. Here's why: First, organic foods aren't always that much more expensive. Some of the cost depends on where you shop. (I'm certainly not planning to do my food shopping on the Upper East Side any time soon.) Second, while you may sometimes spend more on an *individual item*—an organic grapefruit typically costs more than the chemically grown one—you'll spend less on your *overall diet*. Sure, if you choose a bag of organic potato chips, not typical ones, you'll dole out more. But compare organic potatoes with a bag of Ruffles, and now you're talking (see page 98 for a sample day-in-the-life cost comparison).

Sometimes the upfront cost of Grub items can be more than their industrial counterparts. Part of the reason is that it often costs more to grow food organically. There is less infrastructure for distribution, fewer economies of scale, and, except for a handful of cost-sharing programs in some states, no government subsidies to support farmers making the transition to organic or help them out once they do. They've got other things stacked against them, too. Organic growers have to pay five percent more for crop insurance, but if disaster strikes are only compensated at the price level of industrial food, not the organic premium, according to the Organic Farming Research Foundation. Then, there's labor. Organic farms are often labor-intensive and considering that most large-scale industrial operations pay far below a living wage, the small-scale organic farmers who pay their workers fairly can have significantly higher costs.

Here are some ideas for making the Grub diet more affordable.

EAT IN

Today we spend nearly half of our total annual food budget on food away from home, up from one-quarter nearly fifty years ago.[2] Cutting out a few of these away-from-home meals can mean big savings.

WASTE NOT, WANT NOT

You'd be surprised how much money you could save if you paid attention to your garbage. The average household throws away 14 percent of what they spend on food, adding up to nearly $600 a year, according to a University of Arizona study.[3] Most of us don't even realize we do. Said one of the researchers: "It was so bizarre to have people standing there telling you they waste *zero* food, while they're dumping a big platter of spaghetti and meatballs into the garbage!"

BRAND-FREE, BULK OUT

If it's got a brand on it, you're paying for it, literally, with a big chunk of your dollar going to marketing. If your local stores don't carry bulk foods, try asking them to. For items that keep well, you can also save by buying large volumes and decanting them into smaller containers.

When we think of the cost of organic food items, we can think of Sandra Steingraber, scientist, cancer survivor, and author, who says, "I consider buying organic my family's philanthropy." Or the school garden teacher in California who told me she sees her healthy diet as a form of health insurance.

Or, we can think of John Kinsman's words. Kinsman, a Wisconsin organic dairy farmer and founder of Family Farm Defenders, who has been farming for decades, likes to say, "Every time you spend money on food, you are voting for the world you want."

When you vote for real, though, you know who you're voting for, right? At least you see their name on the ballot. But when you shop at a supermarket, the name of the farmer isn't usually on that apple you buy, or the milk you purchase. No, at a typical store with a typical purchase, we don't have that much control over what our dollar "vote" endorses. For every dollar we spend at a typical supermarket, the farmer gets less than two dimes—and still must shoulder all their expenses.[4] Most of our food dollar isn't going to the workers and meat packers who processed our food, or to the workers at the grocery store where we buy it, either. Most of that dollar goes to packaging, transport, and marketing, and into the pockets of the CEOs and agribusiness big whigs.

So how can you have more control over your vote when you shop for food?

Doing a community food audit is the first step to ensuring you're voting your values when you buy your food.

SUP'R STORE MARKET
BROOKLYN, NY

BREAKFAST
```
  BOWL OF BRAND NAME CEREAL    $0.36
  MILK FOR CEREAL              $0.25
  GRAPEFRUIT                   $0.67
  GLASS OF ORANGE JUICE        $0.44
  SUBTOTAL:                    $1.72
```

DELI LUNCH
```
  TURKEY SANDWICH              $4.75
  BIG GRAB BAG OF CHIPS        $0.99

  20 OZ SODA                   $1.25
  SUBTOTAL:                    $6.99
```

SNACK (VENDING MACHINE)
```
  TRAIL MIX                    $0.75
  SODA                         $1.25
  SUBTOTAL:                    $2.00
```

TAKE-OUT DINNER
```
  SM HOT AND SOUR SOUP         $1.65
  BEEF VEGETABLE RICE          $8.25
  SUBTOTAL:                    $9.90
```

DESSERT
```
  OREO COOKIES                 $0.29
  GLASS OF MILK                $0.25
  SUBTOTAL:                    $0.54
```
```
  ------------------------
  GRAND TOTAL:                $21.15
```

‡‡‡‡‡‡THANK YOU‡‡‡‡‡‡‡‡

THE GRUB COOP
BROOKLYN, NY

BREAKFAST
```
  BOWL OF HOMEMADE GRANOLA     $0.24
  ORGANIC YOGURT               $0.78
  ORGANIC RED GRAPEFRUIT       $0.75
  GLASS OF ORGANIC ORANGE JUICE $0.62
  SUBTOTAL:                    $2.39
```

LUNCH
```
  HUMMUS & AVOCADO SANDWICH    $1.75
  (W/LETT ORG TOMATO ONION)
  ORGANIC APPLE                $0.62
  WATER WITH ORGANIC LEMON     $0.05
  SUBTOTAL:                    $2.42
```

SNACK
```
  BANANA                       $0.58

  CUP OF ORGANIC TEA           $0.15
  SUBTOTAL:                    $0.78
```

GRUB DINNER
```
  HOT AND SOUR SOUP            $2.29
  (W/SHIITAKE MUSHROOM)

  SENSUAL VEGETABLE STIR-FRY   $2.31
  (W/RICE)

  SUBTOTAL:                    $4.60
```

DESSERT
```
  BOWL OF ORGANIC ICE CREAM    $0.66
  CUP OF ORGANIC TEA           $0.15
  SUBTOTAL:                    $0.81
```
```
  ------------------------
  GRAND TOTAL:                $10.95
```

The Cost of Food: A Day in the Life of Two Eaters

Prices reflect serving size from package. All "Sup'R" food bought from a large mainstream supermarket unless noted. All "Grub" food bought at a local food cooperative.

STEP 2: GET ON THE RIGHT BUS: COMMUNITY FOOD AUDIT

Keep track of your Community Food Audit with the worksheet on page 331.

We may want to get off the bus—to make different choices about our food—but some of us may not have a clue how to do it or what resources our community has to help us. With your audit, you'll find opportunities for choosing Grub in your own backyard; you may be surprised by how many you have. Your audit will also give you hands-on suggestions about how to transform your neighborhood, city, or region from a food desert into an oasis of healthy choices.

Your audit may also help you for the same reason it helped me: truth is, I can be lazy and weak-willed. Shopping at a typical supermarket, you need determination and diligence to weed the good foods from the bad. Making smart decisions about *where* you shop may be the most important decision of all.

Audit Part 1: Shop Here

FARMERS' MARKETS AND FARMSTANDS

Maybe you have one near your house or apartment and don't even know it. With nearly 4,000 of them across the country and new ones popping up all the time, you can now find farmers' markets in hundreds of cities. In New York City—not exactly everyone's image of farm-fresh food heaven—a quarter of a million people every week pass through the city's forty-seven markets, found in all five boroughs. Nearly half of them operate year-round, even in bristly East Coast winters.

Beginning a decline in the 1920s, farmers' markets reached their lowest point in the 1970s, when there were fewer than one hundred.[5] But in the past decade they've seen a revival, doubling since the mid-1990s.[6] Most farmers' markets are growers' markets, meaning that to sell at them you have to grow the food, too. While the prices may be higher than your local grocery store's, you definitely know where your money is going—you're placing your dollar into their hands. Plus, nothing beats the freshness of the food.

Starting a Farmers' Market: If you can't find a farmers' market near you, visit World Hunger Year's website for tips about starting your own (worldhungeryear.org). You can start small; the Lower East Side Girls Club did. Their farmers' market started in 2003 with one farmer in one of the city's poorest neighborhoods. Now every Saturday in the summer the market brims with life, with Girls Club members helping staff the farmstand, munching on organic fruit, and chatting with customers.

Organic Foods at Farmers' Markets: If you don't see a sign that says "organic," ask the farmer. You may find they're transitioning to organic production, during which time they are not allowed to label their products organic, even though they are forgoing chemicals. Or you may find that they've chosen not to become USDA-certified even though they're eschewing chemicals on the farm.

COMMUNITY SUPPORTED AGRICULTURE FARMS (CSAS)

"If CSAs didn't exist, we wouldn't be here," said Dave Perkins, who farms seventeen organically certified acres with his wife and family near Madison, Wisconsin. Like the thousands of CSA members across the country, their 800 members are "shareholders" in the farm, paying a flat fee upfront to receive fresh food throughout the harvest season. The Perkinses have partnered with area farmers to offer not only produce, but also eggs, meat, even goat cheese. The Perkins also provide their city-locked members occasions to visit the farm, in annual U-pick festivals, corn boils, pesto fests, and pumpkin-picking parties.

CSAs were brought to the United States in 1984, inspired by similar efforts in Japan and Germany. They've expanded exponentially ever since, to more than 1,200 today. Even in ultra-urban New York City you can find dozens of CSAs. As the Perkinses learned, CSAs make farming viable for small producers by guaranteeing customers and supplying essential capital just when farmers need it. In return, members have the assurance of fresh food from farmers they know.

Cost: Some CSAs offer a sliding scale or payment plans if you're unable either to pay the full amount or pay it in one fell swoop. Some nonprofit community organizations also offer cost-sharing to offset the costs.

Starting a CSA: You don't need to be a farmer to start a CSA. Many CSAs are initiated by communities who seek out land and a farmer. Many faith-based organizations are getting in on the act, too, with "congregation-supported agriculture." Contact the Robin Van Eyn CSA Center to learn about starting a CSA (csacenter.org).

FOOD COOPERATIVES

Walk into the Park Slope Food Coop in Brooklyn any day of the week and the place will be bustling with checkout worker/filmmakers and produce stocker/teachers, teeming with cashier/lawyers and custodian/massage therapists. Managed by a core staff, the Coop is run by its 12,000-plus members who, along with their "real" jobs, work a few hours a month as a requirement of membership. (Not every coop requires you to work to be a member.) Like hundreds of other food coops around the country, the Park Slope Food Coop is able to keep its prices low because it does not charge the markups that chain stores do. Because coops don't demand slotting allowances and other fees that make it challenging (if not impossible) for small companies to get onto your shelves, they also can offer more variety and local products.

BUYING CLUBS

Another low-cost strategy, buying clubs are less formal than coops. They don't require a physical store; instead, collectives of friends or community members buy in bulk from distributors, driving down what each individual pays. To learn about starting either, contact the Cooperative Grocer (cooperativegrocer.coop).

RESTAURANTS WITH FARMERS AT HEART

At L'Etoile in Madison, Wisconsin, you can dine in view of a regional map of the local farmers who grew your plate of squash or peas or beans. At the Farmers Diner in Barre, Vermont, all the food—from the beef in the hamburgers to the milk in the milkshakes—comes from local farmers. At Ici Restaurant, a block away from my apartment, you can order Added Value Mixed Greens, imported all the way from Red Hook, Brooklyn, a few miles away. Find out about local restaurants that have jumped on board to source their food locally, and encourage your neighborhood restaurants to do so. One support network for chefs is the ten-year-old Chefs Collaborative, with a membership of 1,100 chefs and farmers (chefscollaborative.org).

Audit Part 2: Look for These Campaigns and Labels

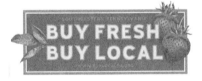

Buy Fresh, Buy Local

A Wisconsin farmer told me about visiting a supermarket chain near Houston, Texas. Above their produce, a sign read "Support your local farmers!" next to a full-color glossy of a smiling farmer. Only one problem: the picture was of him. Yes, he's a farmer, but in Wisconsin—more than a thousand miles away. So how do you know what's local, for real? The folks at FoodRoutes Network based in rural Pennsylvania have been helping those of us who want to choose local by promoting the "Buy Fresh, Buy Local" campaign in nearly a dozen regions across the country. Local groups coordinate and customize the campaign for their region—developing creative strategies to promote local food through a range of direct marketing outlets including CSAs, farmers' markets, restaurants, and farmstands as well as institutions and independently owned grocery stores. To learn more about campaigns in your area, or to start one, contact FoodRoutes (foodroutes.org).

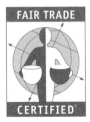

Fair-Trade Certified

Not everything you eat (or drink) can be grown locally. But trace that dollar (or two or three) you spend on your morning coffee fix, and by the time your money has made its way back to the farmer only a few cents, if that, are left. That's where fair-trade certified products come into the picture. Described in Chapter Four, fair-trade certified options now abound, from coffee and tea to chocolate and fruit. Look for them with this label in your grocery stores, cafés, or restaurants. Many churches, schools, hospitals, even city councils are now fair-trade-coffee-only zones.

Fair-Trade on Campus: If you're a student or administrator, contact United Students for Fair Trade (usft.org) or Global Exchange (globalexchange.org) to find out how to bring fair-trade products to your campus.

Audit Part 3: Grow Your Own

The most direct (and cheapest) way to get food you can trust is to grow your own. But grow your own . . . in a city?! In Singapore, 80 percent of the city's poultry and one-quarter of its vegetables come from farms within the city limits.[7] One-fifth of Londoners reportedly grow home gardens; one-half of folks in Vancouver do—two cities that wouldn't be the first on my list of places with perfect weather for farming.[8] The American Community Gardening Association estimates roughly 18,000 community gardens can now be found in the United States; two-thirds grow produce.[9] These figures don't even include the home gardens hidden behind fences and tucked into backyards. You can start small—growing basil in a pot in your window—or find a community garden (or start one) in your neighborhood.

You can also find out about community groups creating grow-your-own opportunities. On Chicago's South Side, a thick-aired greenhouse in the Woodlawn neighborhood just south of Hyde Park houses a spin-off from the Milwaukee-based Growing Power, doing just that. Headed by Erika Allen, a thirty-three-year-old African-American food justice activist, community food systems planner, and aspiring urban farmer, whose father founded the first Growing Power in Milwaukee, the Chicago spin-off is helping bring healthy food into urban communities.

"We're thinking about the whole cycle: how you bring food into a community, and once it's there how it is being consumed so that stays in that community," said Erika, surrounded by five-gallon buckets to be distributed in the community for composting and by hundreds of seedlings bursting out of their plastic cartons. These seedlings will eventually be planted in nearby vacant lots. Harvested by the community—from young kids to elders—they will be a far cry from the Food Emporium's $2.97 organic grapefruit.

Erika's project is just one of hundreds around the country improving food access by teaching farming techniques and building neighborhood networks. To find out more, visit growingpower.org and foodsecurity.org.

Relish Your Rubbish: Just because you live in a city doesn't mean you have to throw away all of your food scraps; you, too, can compost. Here are some options: If you've got a community garden near you, toss food scraps into a bag in your freezer and bring it down to your local garden. (Why the freezer? Because a scrap container on your counter can get gross.) Alternatively, turn to the worms. Keep a vermicompost bin beneath your sink and let worms turn your food waste into rich soil for your houseplants, window boxes, or thankful neighbors. Some cities also have composting programs. Find out if your city is among them—if not, maybe you can help bring composting to town!

Audit Part 4: Get Feisty

Okay, so what if you've gotten this far in the audit and have turned up mostly empty-handed? This is where a little resourcefulness comes in. Most store managers or restaurant owners never hear from their customers—ever. A few queries or suggestions—a little consumer muscle—can go a long way. It's a lot easier than you might think.

A colleague got a phone call from a harried manager of a supermarket near San Francisco. The manager said he'd been bombarded with requests for fair-trade coffee, and was looking for advice about how to find it. After getting off the phone, our friend contacted the folks who had been campaigning at the store and asked what had so ruffled the manager's feathers. "Uh, we sent a dozen postcards," they said, assuming they hadn't done much at all. Well, apparently they had done just enough.

Find out about groups working to bring Grub into your community and link up with others to gain leverage. Learn more from the Organic Consumers Association (organic consumers.org).

If you don't have a group locally, you can also go it alone. It may feel awkward at first, but try asking the manager of your local store or restaurant:

- What local foods do they carry?
- What organic products do they have?
- What fair-trade products do they stock?
- What non-GMO products do they sell?

If their answer is "none, none, none, and none," warmly suggest they carry these products and offer to share reasons why they should and how they can. For ideas about talking with food buyers, visit sustainabletable.org.

STEP 3: PREP SCHOOL

Now it's time to turn to your kitchen. You may find it is collecting cobwebs and critters, or maybe it is ready to go. Either way, here are ideas for making your kitchen a place you'd actually want to cook in (imagine that!). As I worked on this section, I stayed up until two in the morning, prepping my own kitchen. The next morning, I awoke to a gleaming—and pleasant-to-cook-in—kitchen.

Clear It Out, Clean It Up, and Lighten Up

GET RID OF THE DEAD WEIGHT

As a rule of thumb, if you haven't used a pot or a pan or certain silverware for a few years, chances are you won't ever use them. Stash these space-taking extras, and if after a few more months you're still not using them, give them away to charity. (A kitchen stocked with too many of the wrong things is almost as inconvenient as an unstocked kitchen.)

THROW AWAY OLD SPICES

When you buy spices, try to buy small amounts so they don't sit unused for too long. Most chefs recommend throwing out spices after six months, and certainly after a year. We like to use the smell test: spices should be fragrant. If they're not, they've lost their pizzazz.

FENG SHUI YOUR KITCHEN

Okay, so I'm no feng shui expert, but when it comes to your kitchen be sure that the items (spices, utensils, pots, and pans) that you use most often are conveniently arranged. Spend some time making your space user-friendly.

CLEAN YOUR APPLIANCES

Oven: No need to rely on toxic oven cleaners; a little warm water and baking soda will do the trick.

Fridge: If it's anything like mine, you may find a few landmines of old food in its nooks and crannies. Clear out aging food and condiments, and get a fresh box of baking soda to trap odors.

Freezer: You'll want to use every square inch of your freezer, so if you need to, defrost it and get rid of any old items.

Keep On Keepin' On

BE A NEAT FREAK
Dirty dishes in the sink will definitely dis-inspire you from cooking. If you keep your kitchen clean, whenever you want to start cooking, your kitchen will be ready, too.

CLEANING YOUR TOOLS AND SURFACES
Ongoing kitchen hygiene is vital: wash your sponges in the dishwasher (if you have one) every so often, and replace them on a regular basis. If you eat meat, make sure to designate a cutting board just for meat; and wash your knives (and hands) immediately after handling.

CLEANING YOUR FRUITS AND VEGETABLES
Always wash your produce well, especially if you buy chemically grown food. Over-the-counter fruit and vegetable washes are basically bogus, says Consumer Union's Urvashi Rangan. It is just as effective to use diluted vinegar in water.

STEP 4: GET IN GEAR

Don't believe the hype: you definitely don't need lots of bells and whistles to cook healthy meals. A working stove, fridge, sink, and a few essential tools are about all you need. As you review our suggestions, think of these tools as investments. Choose well, care for them, and you'll have them for a lifetime.

Utensils 'R Us: Make sure you have a good set of utensils, such as kitchen tongs, a wooden spoon, a spatula, and a pair of kitchen scissors. Other basic utensils include measuring cups and spoons and the all-important kitchen timer, preferably with multiple timers to help you keep track of several dishes at once.

In the Cut: Get several cutting boards for different uses. If you eat meat and seafood, designate one for prepping it only. Also, keep a separate cutting board just for fruit. Wood tends to hold less bacteria than plastic, but be sure to wash and dry it immediately after using it. To make your wooden cutting board last longer, dab it with oil after drying.

How Hot Is It? A lot of ovens aren't accurate (especially ones in old Brooklyn apartments), so an oven thermometer is a good idea. Think of this as a big money saver: you don't have to buy a new oven!

The Knives Have It: Investing in good knives will make all the difference in your cooking. See if you can try cutting with them before buying them. "A knife is like a tennis racket; you've got to feel comfortable with it," says Didi Emmons, author of *Entertaining for a Veggie Planet*. A good, sharp knife is also a safe knife. If you're able to make precision cuts easily, you're less apt to cut yourself.

A note on knife care: Always store your knives in a block or on a magnetic strip. Never put them in a dishwasher and never cut on a surface that's harder than the knife. Wash and dry your knives immediately after using them. Regularly sharpen them with a knife sharpener, and get them professionally sharpened on occasion.

Slicing, Dicing, and Peeling: Have a hardy peeler to tackle a range of peels and skins, from carrots to winter vegetables to mangoes. You might want a Y-shaped peeler, too, for tough peels. For fancy peels and thin slices, invest in a mandoline slicer. (A good food processor will come with attachments for these thin, creative cuts and grating.)

The Almighty Salad Spinner: This deserves special mention because it is essential if you ever want to eat salad, which we suggest you do—often.

Appliances 'R Us: A lot of the latest gadgets are overrated, but a few appliances are helpful:

- *Blender and/or Food Processor:* If possible, have both. A blender helps create the right texture for creamy soups and smoothies; a food processor enables a range of chopping and blending.
- *Pressure Cooker:* Bring it out of the closet (or your parents' attic)! One friend still uses his mother's: a wedding present from 1947. While typically used for cooking rice, they can cook all kinds of vegetables, fast: thirty-five minutes (or less) for dried beans; five to ten for artichokes; five for winter squash.

A note on microwaves: If you don't already have one, don't feel compelled to buy one. I have lived without a microwave my whole life and feel good that I haven't added another used one to a landfill somewhere.

Recycling your appliances: Visit GreenerChoices.org to learn about ways to recycle your old appliances.

Cookbooks: Having a few essential cookbooks is like having a dictionary or an encyclopedia on your shelf (that is, before the advent of the Internet).

- *The New Whole Foods Encyclopedia,* by Rebecca Wood. Includes buying and cooking tips and a general overview of whole foods, grains, vegetables, and seeds. It also includes both Western and ayurvedic nutritional properties of foods.
- *Diet for a Small Planet* (20th anniversary edition), by Frances Moore Lappé. Still a great resource for understanding the root causes of hunger and how our everyday food choices have global ripples. It also includes recipes for simple vegetarian meals.
- *The New Joy of Cooking,* by Irma S. Rombauer. The bible of cookbooks, it is an indisputable resource for making your way around most ingredients in your kitchen.

The Right (Storage) Stuff: Storing your food well will save you shopping time and help you waste less food.

- *Oils and Spices:* Keep them in cool, dry, dark places: heat, air, and light are their nemeses. Consider keeping spice jars in a drawer and store oil and vinegar in dark glass.
- *Containers and Bags:* Use Ziploc-style bags of all sizes for freezer storage (you can reuse them by rinsing and drying them after using). For leftovers, have on hand a bunch of Tupperware-style containers of multiple sizes.
- *Jars:* Putting grains, flour, pasta, nuts, and herbs in air-tight jars will help your food stay fresh and free of pantry moths.

- *Plastic Be Gone:* While some plastic bottles, containers, and plastic wraps may be harmless, studies have shown that certain plastics (particularly soft plastics) can leach hormone-disrupting chemicals.[10] Don't microwave food covered with plastic wrap or in plastic containers (try covering with wax paper instead). You can use wax paper for wrapping lunch sandwiches, too.

STEP 5: STOCK UP

A well-stocked kitchen needs the right tools as well as essential food items to help you easily make your favorite recipes, snacks, and quick meals. You'll also be able to grab your favorite cookbook and spontaneously create new dishes, since you'll have many of the ingredients you'll need. Add and subtract items from our list to develop your own personalized reserve.

Beans/Legumes: Choose a variety of dried beans—black, black-eyed peas, chickpeas, lentils, pintos, split peas, and kidneys. You have more control over the taste and consistency with dried beans. If you choose canned, be sure to look at the sodium content.

Citrus: When they're in season, we like to have a bowl of lemons and limes to add to recipes and to tall glasses of water.

Herbs and Spices: Your spice rack is your kitchen's foundation. Along with sea salt and whole peppercorns, stock these commonly used spices. Seek out spices that are labeled organic. Also, look for bulk spices, which are cheaper and allow you to buy small amounts at a time to keep your spices fresh.

BASIL*	CUMIN	RED PEPPER FLAKES
CAYENNE PEPPER	NUTMEG (WHOLE SEEDS)	ROSEMARY*
CINNAMON	PAPRIKA	THYME*

* Choose dried when fresh herbs aren't available (1 teaspoon dried for every tablespoon of fresh).

Spices from selected cuisines if you cook these types of foods often:

SOUTH AMERICAN	INDIAN	MEDITERRANEAN	ASIAN
ANNATTO SEED	CARDAMOM	BASIL	STAR ANISE
CHIPOTLE	CORIANDER	CINNAMON	BLACK SESAME SEEDS
CINNAMON	CUMIN	MARJORAM	
SAFFRON	FENNEL	MINT	
RED CHILE POWDER	GARAM MASALA	PARSLEY	
	MUSTARD SEEDS		
	TURMERIC		

Oils: For most cooking, **olive oil** is the best. **Extra-virgin olive oil** is the least processed and has a strong flavor. Use a high-quality extra-virgin for salads and dips and a less expensive variety for cooking. Many ethnic dishes call for nut or seed oils, but unless you cook with these often, don't buy large quantities; they can go rancid quickly. You might also want a neutral-flavored oil, such as canola or grapeseed, which has a lower flashpoint than olive oil, making it better for frying and cooking at high heat. (Look for non-GMO canola; it's your only assurance the oil isn't genetically modified.)

Pastas: Pasta can be part of a well-balanced diet, especially if you choose whole-grain pasta. "I serve whole-wheat pasta to my daughter," said one friend. "I just don't tell her, and she never knows the difference."

Pepper: We recommend **whole black peppercorns** and a good pepper grinder.

Produce: Stock your kitchen with staple produce that will last, like onions, garlic, and potatoes. Store them in a cool, dry place.

Rice: We like to have a variety for different cuisines, at least one **basmati** and one **brown rice.**

Salt: The best way to minimize your salt intake is to stay away from fast food and processed foods. If you're doing the cooking, you control how much salt you use. Plus, salt added while you're cooking helps release the dormant flavors of your food. Use unrefined, **coarse sea salt** for most dishes and **fine sea salt** for baking. We prefer sea salt because it tastes better than standard table salt and is better for you, containing over eighty minerals and aiding in digestion. Experiment with the amount you use; sea salt tends to be stronger than conventional. Taste often. There's a fine line between perfect and ruined.

Soup Stock: Keep organic stock on hand so you can whip up a soup whenever the spirit moves you, especially when you've got vegetables you don't want to waste. Homemade soup is a healthier choice, too. Canned soups tend to contain loads of salt; it's a cheap way for food companies to spike the flavor. (In one 14-ounce can I bought—without consulting the label— I would have gotten 90 percent of my recommended maximum daily intake of sodium!)

Sweeteners: Explore better-for-you sweeteners than refined white sugar, such as honey, maple syrup, and raw cane sugar, to name a few. You'll find that as you cut out refined sugar and high-fructose corn syrup your taste buds will change and appreciate foods that are less sweet.

Canned Tomatoes and Tomato Sauce: If you're feeling adventurous, buy in-season tomatoes and make a sauce to store in your freezer or to can for the winter. (A helpful book on canning and storing foods is *Putting Food By* by Janet C. Greene.)

Vinegar: If you want to kick up the flavor of most dishes, you need to add some acid. This can come in the form of fresh citrus fruits, such as lemons and limes or bottled vinegars. We like to keep on hand **apple cider** and **balsamic vinegars.** You might also want to stock up on **red and white wine vinegars** and **brown rice vinegar.** Experiment and find the vinegars you like best.

STEP 6: TIME-SAVING TRICKS

Cooking doesn't have to take half your day, or all your evening. Here are some suggestions for saving shopping and cooking time. Look for more tips dabbled throughout Bryant's recipes.

Embrace Your Inner (Liberated) Chef

One of the best time-saving tips is to get familiar (if you're not already) with some cooking basics. Using recipes in our book—or any good cookbook—learn how to make your favorite basic dishes. Once you've got them under your belt, you can start cooking these dishes *sans* recipe, with tweaks for your own taste and with ingredients you happen to have available.

Your Freezer Is Your Friend

Maximizing your freezer's potential will help you waste less food. Says one chef about hers: "My freezer is my oasis. It's my storage bin: nuts, bread, sliced coconut, spring roll wrappers, fruit for smoothies, sturdy herbs. My freezer has 150 things in it."

- **Bread:** If you don't make it through a whole loaf quickly, no need for half to go stale. Buy fresh bread, slice it, and store it in the freezer.
- **Herbs:** When Bryant heads to the farmers' market he always gets an extra bunch of basil. When he gets home he'll wash and dry it and make a paste with oil that he'll freeze to use later in sauces, soups, and other dishes. Sturdy herbs, like rosemary, sage, oregano, or marjoram, can be stored directly in your freezer.
- **Leftovers:** Use portion-size containers, so you defrost only what you want. For concentrated sauces, like pesto, freeze the sauce in an ice cube tray.

Cook for Two (or Three, or Four, or Five)

They say to eat for two when you're pregnant, but no need to be pregnant to cook for two or more. Consider doubling (or tripling or quadrupling) your meals and saving leftovers for lunches or snacks.

Think Ahead

We may have the best intentions when we buy fresh produce, but sometimes it still ends up forgotten and wilted at the back of the fridge. Try prepping your veggies as soon as you get home. With lettuces, for instance, cut, wash, and dry them. Then, wrap loosely in a linen towel (or place in a bag) and store in the fridge. With veggies like broccoli or kale, steam or sauté them as soon as they arrive home. They'll last longer and will more likely be eaten. With fresh herbs, trim the bottoms, and store standing in a bottle with a little water. Cover with a plastic bag and change the water every couple of days.

KNOW WHAT TO DO WITH WHAT YOU GET

Be sure to put produce in all the right places. For mushrooms, store in a paper bag. For onions and potatoes and other vegetables that don't need refrigeration, put them in a cool, dry, dark place. Store ripe whole tomatoes at room temperature.

SNACK RIGHT

Sometimes you don't have time to cook a full meal, or just want a fast bite. This is when the food industry gets us with their tempting "Five Minutes Or Less!" promises of quick sustenance. But we can choose homemade alternatives that are often cheaper, healthier, and just as quick. Microwave popcorn, for instance, often contains added not-good-for-you fats, like partially hydrogenated palm oil or other partially hydrogenated oil, and is loaded with salt. With homemade popcorn, you control the amount of oil and salt. Juice is often loaded with added high-fructose corn syrup, with calories you often don't notice. Nonorganic juice will also load you up with pesticide residues, while actual organic fruit is, well, just fruit. Here are some more examples of the less expensive and better-for-you Grub choice.

THE EXPENSIVE CHOICE	THE GRUB CHOICE
MICROWAVE POPCORN	HOMEMADE POPCORN
STORE-BOUGHT FRUIT JUICE	ACTUAL FRUIT
CANDY BAR	HOMEMADE TRAIL MIX
STORE-BOUGHT CEREAL	HOMEMADE GRANOLA
POTATO CHIPS	RICE CAKES

STEP 7: YOUR ORGANIC LIFE

Since we come into contact with toxics throughout our lives, not just in our food, this step offers tips to cultivate an organic *life*—not just an organic kitchen.

KNOW YOUR H$_2$O

A friend recently asked for tap water at a train station's concession stand. "Tap water, what's that?" the cashier answered, genuinely perplexed. Ah, yes, remember the quaint old days when we got our water from faucets? Unless you've been living in a cave for the past ten years, you'll know bottled water is now big business, spurred on in part by real concerns about our water supply. In a 2002 study, the U.S. Geological Survey found one or more chemicals—including human and veterinary drugs, natural and synthetic hormones, and insecticides—in 80 percent of the sampled streams.[11] Another study found that millions of Americans have been drinking municipal water contaminated at levels far greater than may be safe with chemical by-products from chlorine, which has been linked to miscarriages and birth defects, possibly some cancers, immune system problems, and other illnesses.[12] But inside those bottles with high-design labels and clever copy, the water is not necessarily any "cleaner." Bottled water regulations don't necessarily ensure either purity or safety. Instead of paying between 240 and 10,000 times more per gallon of bottled water for its veneer of safety we can pressure our elected officials to ensure public water supplies are truly safe and clean.[13] After all, access to clean water, like that to healthy food, should be a human right. To learn about your water supply and support policy to protect it, visit epa.gov/safewater and find out about your local water utility at epa.gov/safewater/dwinfo.

SCRUB-A-DUB

Washing your hands may go without saying, but here's another reason to abide by this advice: studies have shown that synthetic chemicals can vaporize and settle on surfaces in our homes—counters, tables, furniture, clothes—surfaces that you then touch with your hands.[14] Washing them frequently will help reduce your exposure.

CUT THE CHEMICALS IN YOUR BOOZE

Thanks to forward-thinking vintners, you can now enjoy a good Shiraz (or Merlot or Chardonnay) without downing wine grapes that were raised with chemicals. Look for organic wines (from France, it's known as *agriculture biologique*), and ask for them at your local wine shop. You can also find organic microbrews, vodka, and other booze, too. If you have a favorite vintner, contact them about making the switch. They can learn from the Lodi-Woodbridge Winegrape Commission in California, for instance, which offers innovative education programs to help farmers get off the chemical treadmill. We'll toast to that!

LOVE YOUR BUGS (KIND OF)

Cockroaches? They're not my favorite critters either, but most home insecticides are highly toxic. Studies have shown links between common household pesticides and birth defects, neurological damage, and the most deadly cancers.[15] Their overuse has also helped create some of the resistant strains of super-bugs we now contend with. Look into nontoxic alternatives. Even better, try prevention: keep a clean house, vacuum often, and bathe your pets frequently.

HOW DOES YOUR GARDEN GROW?

A typical suburban lawn is doused with four to six times the amount of pesticides per acre than farmland, even though landscaping options abound for growing your lawn (and garden) without toxic chemicals.[16] You can shell out hundreds of dollars a year for chemical lawn care; a natural alternative can run you just a fraction of that. For the lawnless urban dwellers among us, we also have nontoxic options for our houseplants. Find out about these resources and more at Beyond Pesticides (beyondpesticides.org).

DON'T PLAY GOLF

Well, you can, but when you're teeing off, keep in mind that golf courses are sprayed with ten times more pesticides per acre than agricultural land.[17] If you are a die-hard enthusiast, talk with your club about using less toxic alternatives. Also, be conscientious about exposure to chemicals on other "greens"—parks, schoolyards, and playgrounds. If you have children, remember the drill: they should wash their hands after playing. If you want to do more, join initiatives in your community to create pesticide-free zones in local parks or schools.

YOUR SKIN IS YOUR LARGEST ORGAN

Cotton uses three to five times more pesticides per acre than corn or soybeans.[18] With increasing consumer demand, more outfitters are offering organic fabric options. Find out if your favorite clothing companies are among them. Look for more information from the Organic Consumers Association (organicconsumers.org).

KISS MY FACE (REALLY)

Skin and body care products come even closer to us than the clothes we wear. As of this writing, the USDA has agreed that cosmetics can display a "certified organic" seal if their ingredients meet the standards. Too bad most cosmetics don't. In fact, many contain potentially toxic ingredients. The government can't even require premarket safety testing of the ingredients that go into our cosmetics. Of the 10,500 chemical ingredients used in personal care products, only 11 percent have been assessed for their safety, according to the Environmental Working Group.[19] Learn more about the chemicals in our cosmetics at ewg.org.

STEP 7½: CELEBRATE

Step 7½ is what this is all comes down to: celebration. Unfortunately, for many of us food has become more and more relegated to something we fear, something we do on the run between home and our office, something to stuff down in front of the evening news. But we human beings have ancient and sacred long-held traditions of eating, of breaking bread together as families, friends, and communities. Let's be part of bringing those traditions back.

When I went online to see what national efforts were being made on this front, I came across this one: "National Eat Dinner Together Week," which calls itself a "salute" to the "tradition of family mealtime." Who can argue with that? Only it turns out the week is a marketing gimmick for "the other white meat." It's a public relations ploy from the Pork Information Bureau, replete with recipes.

To bring back these celebratory food traditions, we prefer Grub parties: intimate, spirited dinners inspired by our love of good food, good conversation, and good wine and music to go along with it.

With Grub parties in mind, Bryant created recipes that make wonderful meals. So cook his delectable menus and throw your own: Invite friends, or strangers. Invite people you've always wanted to have a conversation with; people whom you would never find in a room together. Invite your neighbor. Invite your first crush. Invite your mother. Invite your hero. Be bold.

Our Grub party traditions—the gift, the blessing, the talk, and the closing—add flavor and spirit. Include them, or make up traditions of your own.

The Gift: At our first Grub party, as the snow came pelting down outside Tami's SoHo loft, we had our first taste of the gift exchange. At the beginning of a Grub party we draw names and each person gives a gift to the person whose name they've drawn and describes their gift's significance. That first night, Jee shared *Another World Is Possible,* which he helped conceive, write, and publish within months of 9/11. Adriana gave Jessie cookies in the shape of peace doves with V-O-T-E spelled across them from the Lower East Side Girls Club. Sid passed on a copy of a documentary he produced and Greg rhymed about the connections between the diamond trade, civil war in Africa, and hip-hop bling-bling (before Kanye West, I might add). The gifts were as varied as the guests. By the time we were done, the ice was more than broken—it had thoroughly melted.

The Blessing: In the backyard of a bungalow in West Berkeley, we threw our second Grub party. That evening, as the sun set and the tiki torches lit the overgrown garden, Mike offered a blessing and another friend read a poem before we began the meal. (We've included poems interspersed with the menus for inspiration.) A central part of every Grub meal, the blessing is a moment for reflection before we scarf down the food. We think you'll be surprised by how much better food tastes once you've taken the time to be thankful.

The Talk: At the third Grub party, Bryant invited chef Michele Thorne. As we nibbled on appetizers, Michele talked about the philosophy of raw foods, and guests prodded her with questions, which she patiently answered. You might think about inviting a guest with a particular expertise, or pairing Grub parties with a book club or a film screening.

The Closing/The Beginning: We close each Grub party with a chance for people to thank the hosts, the cooks, and the organizers. It's also a chance for people to exchange contact information. (Already we can count two job offers and one date.)

Those are our traditions; use them, or make up some of your own. And don't forget to save us a place at the table!

SEVEN

Out of the Kitchen, Into the Fire

You hear the thundering *thwack, thwack, thwack* of helicopters. You see copter blades slicing through the nighttime sky above Los Angeles. A light mist of malathion descends over the sleeping city.

The opening images from Robert Altman's 1993 film *Short Cuts* were the perfect representation of our Sisyphean fight against nature. In real life, California had been fighting a losing battle against the dreaded Mediterranean fruit fly, which was threatening the state's citrus fields. Helicopters were sent to blanket its cities in a malathion attack, despite warnings about the public health dangers of the organophosphate pesticide. But those hovering helicopters also represented connection—the connection between the lives of Altman's seemingly disparate twenty-two characters. The helicopters were his reminder that we are all, literally, under the same sky.

In the real world, we might do well to remember the message of those helicopters. We *are* all under the same sky; only sometimes it's harder to see. If it were easier, we could better sense how our choices affect one another, whether you live in the house next door, across town, or across the country.

Of course, for some choices it's pretty easy to see how my actions might affect you: driving safely is obviously good for me, and you. But the effects of our choices to eat Grub are slightly less obvious, even though these decisions have effects that extend far beyond each of us.

Nearly fifty years ago, in her prophetic *Silent Spring,* Rachel Carson wrote that "we stand now where two roads diverge." One road, she said, is "deceptively easy, a smooth superhighway on which we progress with great speed, but at its end lies disaster." The other? It "offers our last, our only chance to reach a destination that assures the preservation of our earth. The choice, after all is ours to make."[1]

Fifty years later we're traveling with increasing velocity in the direction Carson warned of, relying on petroleum- and chemical-addicted farming to bring us our food with damage even she might have been surprised by. But it is still not too late to choose the other road. It's a choice we make every day, multiple times, when we choose whether our food leads us farther along a superhighway of destruction, or not.

And it's a choice we make beyond our consumption decisions: we make it when we choose what to do (or not do) as community members and citizens. Our choices in these spheres hold perhaps the most potential of all. The following stories illustrate this power. Hundreds of similar stories unfold every day. Maybe you will be part of creating the next one.

FOOD U: SHIFTING INSTITUTIONAL PURCHASING AND CHANGING OUR FOOD ECONOMY, ONE MEAL TICKET AT A TIME

"They were forging IDs!" said Josh Viertel of Yale University's Sustainable Food Project, referring not to students faking documents for an over-21 club, but for a campus dining hall promoting sustainable foods.

The idea is, at its heart, simple: university food service is a $4.4 billion a year business, with some small private colleges spending up to $7 million annually.[2] Why not encourage these institutions to channel even a portion of those resources toward Grub—local, organic food from small farmers and from companies who have solid worker-rights records?

While the principle behind farm-to-college is simple, bringing it to life can be complicated.

"Institutions on this scale are used to making one phone call to one supplier for all they need," noted one farm-to-college organizer. "They're used to sourcing from the lowest bidder with food that requires little preparation."

But with a growing demand from students, food service directors, and institutional leaders, colleges are launching farm-to-college programs like wildfire. In the Northeast, Northwest, and Midwest, the number of these programs has doubled in the past ten years. Nationwide you can find more than 200 campuses buying from local farmers in a significant way.[3]

The Yale Sustainable Food Project is one. It started in fall 2003, with one item—apples—in one dining hall.

"That first season, we cleaned out Wayne Young's crop," said Melina Shannon-DiPietro, associate director with Viertel. "We made it possible for Wayne, a fourth-generation farmer, to stay on the land." In a state that loses roughly 8,000 acres of farmland every year, this was no small feat.

Within a year, apples had expanded to a selection of produce; one dining hall had expanded to all thirteen, serving all 4,500 students.

The project has even turned its eye to meat. In 2005, they bought 20,000 pounds of ground beef from a local cooperative of grass-based beef farmers who raise and slaughter their animals humanely.

"We've been to the slaughterhouse where our meat gets processed," Viertel said, "and it's not Eric Schlosser-land," referring to the troubling meatpacking conditions documented in *Fast Food Nation.*

The first question a state inspector asked on a recent visit to the slaughterhouse was "Where's the metal detector?"—a requirement in large processing plants to ensure stray pieces of machinery don't wind up in the meat.

"It's laughable to imagine worrying about that there," said Viertel. "The plant has just two guys; it's clean and calm and safe."

The Yale effort and other farm-to-college projects are discovering the power in connecting with suppliers. They're creating new markets, new products, new possibility. Farmers, for instance, are partnering to form cooperatives to pool their products and organize supply so they can provide schools with the quality, quantity, and consistency needed. Universities are collaborating to buy local, sharing knowledge about channels of supply and demand. Food service providers are communicating with farmers about their needs and developing new production.

This rethinking of cafeteria fare is not restricted to the halls of the Ivy League, or even just to colleges. More than 400 school districts, including some of the nation's largest, spread throughout twenty-three states now buy some food from local farmers, up from only ten a decade ago.[4]

Of course, we still have a long way to go. "The vast majority of what is spent on school meals does not go to fresh fruits and vegetables and certainly not foods from local farmers," stresses chef and author Ann Cooper, one of the nation's leading advocates for school food reform.

But the *potential* is enormous. Imagine if the USDA diverted just a sliver of the roughly $10 billion it spends every year on school lunches and breakfasts and summer food service programs toward farm-fresh food? Imagine how our farming economy, our landscape, and our food options would be changed. A few federal programs do promote local, whole foods: the USDA, for instance, offers the Farmers' Market Nutrition Program for low-income women with children and the Senior Farmers' Market Nutrition Program for low-income seniors, but the vouchers range from $10 to $40 for the entire year.[5] Better than nothing, but you can't buy a whole lot of anything with the equivalent of a dollar or two a month. The Department of Defense's Fresh Produce program also supports small family farmers by buying local, fresh produce for schools, hospitals, and prisons in forty-three states. In 2004, the program channeled $74 million to farmers, a big jump from its first-year total of roughly $3 million ten years earlier.[6]

Shifting institutional buying also does more than just improve health. "It contributes to enlightenment," said the founder of a farm-to-school program in Michigan, "helping kids understand that Lunchables aren't one of the food groups; that chicken isn't a square breaded fried nugget."

Whether we are parents of children in public schools, administrators at a hospital or a university, or members of community groups or churches, we can think about shifting institutional food buying choices. (Imagine Sunday services with carrots and local apples and fair-trade coffee, instead of donuts and instant coffee?)

Yale's Josh Viertel put it this way when he described the social significance of these efforts. Referring to the abysmal conditions in Upton Sinclair's muckraking classic, he said, "Students shouldn't be reading *The Jungle* in English 101, and then going and eating it for lunch!" None of us should.

DAVID VS. GOLIATH AND SOMETIMES DAVID WINS: CITIZENS SHAPE POLICY

No county in the country had ever done it before. But when Mendocino County residents in Northern California went to the voting booths on March 2, 2004, the citizens passed a measure to prohibit the raising of genetically modified crops and animals there.

The win for Measure H was not for lack of industry trying. In this small agricultural county of 47,000 voters, the industry-funded "Citizens Against Measure H" poured more than half a million dollars into blocking the measure.

While the group may sound like a coalition of county residents, it was mainly the pooled resources of biotech companies, including CropLife America, DuPont, Dow, and Monsanto, one of the leading makers of GMOs. (Monsanto has a long history in the county: in the mid-1990s residents successfully fought against the company's roadside spraying of their herbicide Roundup.)

Who was *for* the measure? A coalition of real farmers and flesh-and-blood citizens concerned about GMOs. The primary concerns centered on the possible contamination of organic farms with genetically modified crops.

"We didn't have GMOs here, yet, so people saw Measure H as a proactive way to protect the environment," said Britt Bailey, a scientist, environmentalist, and county resident who, along with others including my father helped draft the measure's language.

The California (now the Western) Plant Health Association, which represents industrial agriculture in the state, made the first attempt to thwart the measure by filing a lawsuit claiming misleading language in the ballot.[7] At the hearing, held on Christmas Eve 2003, the courtroom was standing room only. During the hearing, the attorney representing Measure H supporters said, look, we have the First Amendment. If opponents to the measure didn't like the ballot language, they could use the rebuttal space in the ballot to say so.[8]

The language in the ballot remained. The measure went forward, and so did the industry efforts to derail it. For independent-minded Mendocino residents, opposition-funded media pushed all the right buttons. First, industry warned that the measure would raise taxes in enforcement costs. But campaign coordinators let residents know the measure wouldn't cost the county a dime; if it did a volunteer group had already stepped forward, willing to cover the bill.

The opposition also suggested the measure would threaten residents' personal liberties, asking forebodingly: "Does the government need to know what's growing in your garden?" Ironically, the opposite is true: *industry* could be tramping through your backyard, not government. Any farmer who plants genetically modified seeds must sign a technology agreement, which forbids farmers from saving the seeds and replanting them. The agreement also permits the company to survey your farmland to enforce it. "When you plant GMOs, you grant authority to corporate detail people to walk your land for years after you plant to see if you've illegally saved any of their seeds," explained Bailey.

To combat the misinformation, citizens organized dozens of teach-ins and public hearings, on just a fraction of industry's budget. Despite hundreds of thousands of industry dollars, on March 2, 2004, Measure H passed.

While the victory has inspired similar measures in more than half a dozen other counties, it has also led to industry backlash. Within less than a year, fifteen states have introduced legislation that would take away authority of local governments (towns, counties, or municipalities) to make decisions pertaining to seeds, or plants, according to Bailey.

And though two other California counties have passed similar legislation, four others have tried and lost. "Still, these campaigns are part of a global movement," stressed a GE-Free organizer in California. "They are happening around the world, and won't go away."

THE ONE-HUNDREDTH PENCIL

At the end of a recent University of Pennsylvania symposium on buying local foods, Maurice Sampson, a middle-aged man sitting among dozens of college students, raised his hand.

"I don't have a question, exactly," he began, six words that tend to send a wave of fear through any audience during a question-and-answer period. But instead of a long-winded tirade, he offered this powerful story.

In the mid-1990s, Sampson had been working with the city of Philadelphia, which had recently declared a new environmental policy that when possible any city purchase should be from recycled materials.

One day the city received a prototype of a recycled pencil, and though they were slightly more expensive than standard pencils, the city decided the extra cost was worth it.

"That one purchase," Sampson said, "bumped up the manufacturer's economy of scale to a volume at which the price per recycled pencil became equivalent to what you pay for a standard one. The pencils were instantly competitive. As a result of the city's one decision, you can now buy recycled pencils at OfficeMax, Staples, anywhere you want."

As Sampson talked, I thought of the city's decision as the "one-hundredth monkey." Maybe you've heard that phrase, too, used to describe a tipping point. The saying, as I remembered it, comes from the findings of researchers who discovered that monkeys living on a small island sometime in the last century exhibited an amazing trait: once 100 monkeys learned a new technique, suddenly monkeys everywhere caught on and the new skills spread like wildfire.

But then I looked into the story. Though there seems to have been an island, and there was a researcher, even some monkeys, the story, otherwise, is apocryphal.

So maybe it's time to replace that allegory with Sampson's pencils. And the key lesson? Any of our actions, at any moment, could be the one-hundredth pencil. Maybe it's our city council's (or hospital's, or school's) purchase of local carrots that tips our regional food economy so that it can support local farms. Maybe it is campus organizing that convinces a university to boycott its source of meat until the company guarantees workers' rights. Maybe it is one visit or phone call or campaign that tips your local officials to put in place stiffer pesticide regulations. Maybe it's a conversation with a college roommate, who goes on to become CEO of a Fortune 500 food company, that influences him or her to shift the company's buying practices to support organic farming. Maybe it's your decision to join a CSA, visit a farmers' market, or buy from a local food cooperative that staves off the hemorrhaging of farms in your region.

As consumers, we make dozens of decisions about food every day. As citizens and community members, we have endless ways to make a difference. Opportunities abound.

Many of us, though, may not perceive our own power. We worry that any action we may take will be just a drop in that proverbial bucket. Even worse, we fear that we're like drops in the Sahara: our efforts evaporate before even touching ground. For, if we could really sense a bucket, we could see our potential. After all, drops in a bucket add up quite fast.

So what is the bucket? It is all the efforts described here—that you discover when you seek out your community food audit and that you uncover when you learn of the ecological farming revolution, the local food revival, and the emergent food justice movement.

Each time we act, every time we eat, we become part of something much bigger than our individual selves. We're helping to fill the bucket, our drops adding to a global movement toward a more sustainable planet, spurred on by thousands, millions even, of drops just like us.

What if you could really sense this? What if you knew that the investments you made now—in the form of that apple you buy, that farmer you support, that policy you advocate for—would build strong community? What if you knew these choices would have ramifications a generation from now? Would you waver while your hand hovered over that organic apple? Would your feet hesitate on a Saturday morning as you set out to your local farmers' market? In the ballot booth, would your arm linger over the lever for a candidate who endorses agriculture policies that support small, family farms and organic production?

And what if you knew, could really feel it in your bones, how our actions here in the United States have global ripples? What if you could really feel the impact of putting your dollars into the hands of local producers as opposed to contributing to the advertising budgets of multi-national food companies that now spread from the foothills of the Himalayas to the islands of Indonesia? What if you could really sense that every time you bought fair-trade food you helped farmers somewhere in the world feed their own families? Or that every time you bought organic produce you were helping us get off the pesticide treadmill and shift away from addiction to toxic chemicals?

When we make the choice to get on the right bus—to embrace a different relationship to our food, to our economy, to our communities—we never will know all of the people who will be touched, all of the ways our world will be changed. We certainly will never know if any of our actions will be that one-hundredth pencil.

Instead of being disheartened by what we cannot know, we can be liberated by this un-knowing. Liberated, we can surrender to the unknown and take action. The choice is still ours to make.

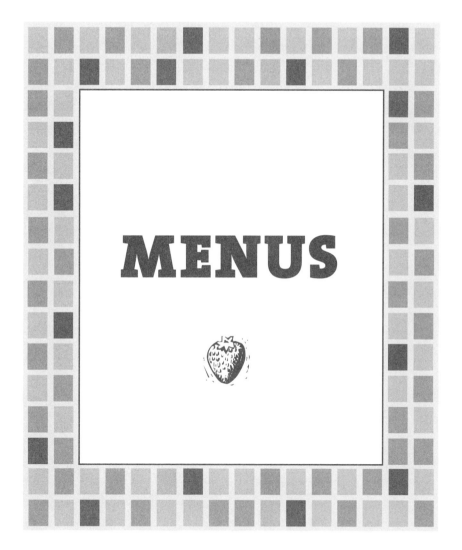

MENUS

What's in Season?

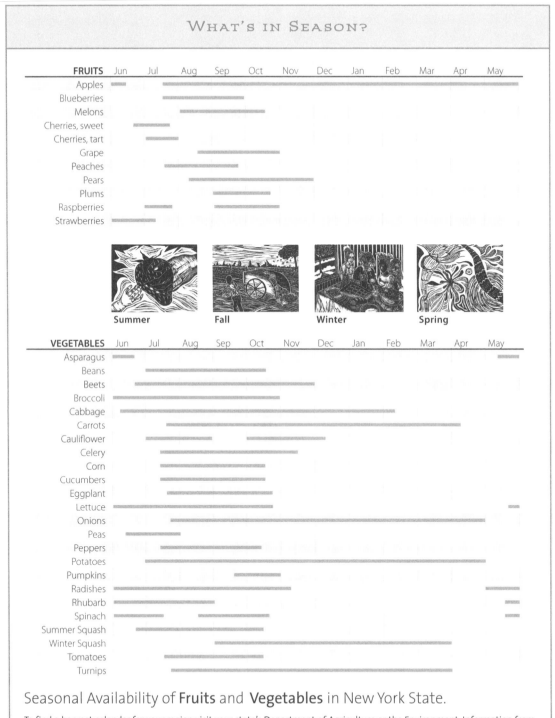

FRUITS	Jun	Jul	Aug	Sep	Oct	Nov	Dec	Jan	Feb	Mar	Apr	May
Apples												
Blueberries												
Melons												
Cherries, sweet												
Cherries, tart												
Grape												
Peaches												
Pears												
Plums												
Raspberries												
Strawberries												

Summer   Fall   Winter   Spring

VEGETABLES	Jun	Jul	Aug	Sep	Oct	Nov	Dec	Jan	Feb	Mar	Apr	May
Asparagus												
Beans												
Beets												
Broccoli												
Cabbage												
Carrots												
Cauliflower												
Celery												
Corn												
Cucumbers												
Eggplant												
Lettuce												
Onions												
Peas												
Peppers												
Potatoes												
Pumpkins												
Radishes												
Rhubarb												
Spinach												
Summer Squash												
Winter Squash												
Tomatoes												
Turnips												

Seasonal Availability of **Fruits** and **Vegetables** in New York State.

To find a harvest calendar for your region visit your state's Department of Agriculture or the Environment. Information from the New York State Department of Agriculture & Markets. Note: Some harvest seasons can be extended.

Getcha Grub On

Diets are dead!

And I am not just referring to the latest get-thin-quick weight-loss schemes. I'm also referring to those rigid labels: Raw Foodist, Fruitarian, Vegan, Lacto-ovo-vegetarian, Lacto-vegetarian, Ovo-vegetarian, Pescetarian, Omnivore . . . the problem is not with these diets, per se; it is with food dogmatism.

When considering health reasons for choosing foods, we needn't always be hard-liners. We all have specific body constitutions, cultural foodways, and personal tastes that determine which foods work for us; no single way of eating is perfect for everyone. In fact, because our bodies are so dynamic, no single diet is perfect for any one of us throughout our life. Our relationship with food should be fluid, shifting as we change.

Zealously embracing dietary models can back us into a corner and prevent us from fully enjoying a healthy relationship with food. This type of rigid thinking was typified in a comment a friend recently made to me: "I would have some of the salad you made, but you sprinkled Parmesan cheese on it." *(In a whisper)* "I actually like Parmesan cheese; it reminds me of my grandmother's Italian cooking, but I don't want to look like a hypocrite, since I'm a vegan." I have heard similar comments from innumerable people. I have seen vegans secretly eating dairy, and vegetarians sneaking seafood. I have even seen die-hard meat eaters enjoying a salad or a veggie burger.

Diet often becomes a role that intimately is tied up in one's identity. For a lot of people, changing diets means reinventing oneself, and that can be understandably complicated (even terrifying). Those striving to eat more healthfully must be brave.

If we did away with artificial boundaries around what we eat, what would eating healthy mean? Ultimately, each individual needs to answer this question by closely examining how certain foods make her or him feel spiritually and emotionally as well as physically. If you feel too heavy from eating meat at every meal, is it really *that* balanced? If you are not enjoying eating that brown rice and tofu with steamed kale, is it really *that* healthy for you? Eating healthfully requires that we move beyond food pyramids and nutrient content and expand our notion of what "healthy eating" really entails. I used to be a food militant, seeing food merely as fuel that I needed in order to be healthy and robust. I lost touch with the joy of eating and soon realized that food should not be utilitarian; it is meant to be enjoyed. Our meals should be healing but should not resemble taking medicine.

Our diets should be spontaneous, flexible, and creative. Living a healthy life is about enjoying each moment and reveling in its magic. Hence, our relationship with food should not be burdensome. Furthermore, healthy food does not have to be bland and tasteless. It can (and should) be delicious. Our meals should strengthen our bodies, lift our spirits, and emotionally ground us.

If you do not have deep-seated ethical issues against eating sustainable dairy, seafood, poultry, beef, or pork occasionally, and if the indulgence makes you feel good, is that act bad? If eating a dessert a few times a week puts a smile on your face, is this really a "sin"? As you will see when you make it, a sweet, rich slice of **Chocolate–Pecan Pudding Pie** can temporarily melt away worries, make you clap your hands, stomp your feet, and scream "hallelujah."

Food should move us to a better place.

The Grub cuisine resists labeling. So when perusing these menus, try not to wrack your brain figuring out what category these fit into and for whom they are intended. I will tell you right now—these recipes are for anyone who loves to eat delicious, healthy, and sustainable *home cooking.* When composing these menus, I primarily used local and seasonal produce from the Northeast. A couple of the menus reinterpret different "ethnic" cuisine and call for ingredients that are not from the Northeast. The majority of the recipes are free of animal products, but a few are whipped up with butter, cheese, eggs, and seafood. Most of the recipes are simple enough for any home chef to make without Emeril Lagasse coaching them through each procedure.

Not everyone may want to prepare all the recipes exactly as written; and that's okay. Use each as a guide. Freestyle and be creative. Consider your (and your guests') personal tastes, desires, ethics, politics, and dietary restrictions when preparing these menus. Feel free to add, omit, or substitute suggested ingredients for those that make more sense for you. For example, if you want to source your meal locally, add the collard greens you got from the farmer down the street to the miso soup in the **Simply Macrobiotic** menu. If you do not eat shellfish, substitute chunks of finfish or tofu for the shrimp in the **Afrodiasporic Cookout** menu. If you do not eat dairy products, leave out the cheese when making the Baby Bella Mushroom Quesadillas in the **¡Grub Latinoamericana!** menu. And if you want to eat meat, substitute chunks of beef chuck for the seitan in that same menu. As Chef Daniel Boulud reminds us, "A recipe, by definition, is never entirely proprietary, [but] ripe for reinterpretation by any creative chef."

Be creative and make these recipes your own.

As you will read in the headnotes, most of these menus have the texture of autobiography, revealing an ever-evolving relationship with food: growing up in Memphis eating my family's soul food (**New Millennium Soul Food** and **New Year's Eve Good Luck Hors d'Oeuvres**); inhaling overstuffed Po Boys and other Cajun/Creole delights while living in New Orleans (**Mardi Gras Grub**); discovering West Indian food in my old New York neighborhood—Crown Heights, Brooklyn (**Ital Grub**); and eating Mexican food in Mexico and San Francisco's Mission District (**Down South of the U.S. Border**).

Other menus are more functional. The **Valentine's Day Decadence** menu was designed to help you titillate your lover (or potential lover), and the **After-Dinner Dessert Buffet** should satisfy your sweet tooth.

The range of menus is our way of demonstrating that Grub does not have to look a certain way. With the use of best-quality ingredients, health-supportive cooking techniques, and your positive energy, a lot of food can be Grub.

We invited friends to contribute menus, too. Lara Comstock Oramas, with whom I started LEFTovers Progressive Catering Company, created a tantalizing **Cuban Comfort** menu that was inspired by her Cuban roots and North American upbringing. Ludie Minaya and Elizabeth Johnson, the backbone of b-healthy's CHOP (Creating Healthy Organic Power) Education and Organizing Project, collaborated on a mouthwatering **Afro-Latina Tapas** menu, which is a confluence of their knowledge of African-American and Latin American foodways. While many of the ingredients in these two spring menus come from other parts of the globe, these culinary delights underscore the importance of constantly renewing our connection with ancestral foods for individual health.

All of the menus are designed with the hope that you will invite a few friends over and have **Grub parties**. Therefore, we invited Katrine Pollari—owner of Olivino Wines in Brooklyn—to provide wine suggestions where appropriate. We certainly are not suggesting that you drink alcohol at every meal (it is high in sugar, ya know), but we want to recommend wines that will complement each menu. And feel free to experiment with different wines to see which ones work best for you, too. As I have said, these menus (and the Grub parties) should express your personality. Whatever you decide to drink, good company is the best accompaniment for this food.

The treats do not rest on the pages alone. Each menu also includes a soundtrack of suggested albums for your aural pleasure—from acid jazz to zydeco. I love music (I even dedicated a menu to hip-hop— **Beets, Limes, and Rice: Salad Selection for Heads**). But instead of recommending all of *my* favorite tunes, we invited friends to suggest music to help you create the right ambiance while you are preparing, cooking, and partying. We also asked a few gifted friends to contribute creative pieces.

There are more treats peppered throughout this section, but I do not want to tell you everything. So, ignore the labels, explore the food, poetry, and music. Shake your booty, and *Getcha Grub On!*

BRYANT TERRY
Oakland, California

- Visit eatgrub.org to get printable shopping lists for each menu.

- Read each menu completely before you start cooking.

- Unless otherwise noted, all menus will serve four to six people and are designed for small dinner parties.

- When making a full menu, save time by prepping ingredients that are common to other recipes all at once. For example, if a main and a side both call for fresh lemon juice, squeeze it all at once.

- Review the time-saving tips following each menu.

- Ask friends and family members to help you prepare meals.

- Although these are complete meals, remember you can prepare any of the recipes on their own.

FROM SEED TO TABLE

We give thanks to all who contribute to meals, from seed to table
To mother earth who bears precious seeds and provides the perfect conditions for growth
To hardworking farmers who plant, care for, and harvest nourishing Grub
To chefs who envision, carefully prepare, and lovingly cook delicious food
We give you thanks

Grub Menus

▪ SUMMER ▪

Down South of the U.S. Border (La Linea)
Ital Grub
Beets, Limes, and Rice: Salad Selection for Heads
Afrodiasporic Cookout
Straight-Edge Punk Brunch Buffet (DIY)

▪ FALL ▪

After-Dinner Dessert Buffet
¡Grub Latinoamericana!
More Than One Side (Dish) to Thanksgiving

▪ WINTER ▪

New Year's Eve Good Luck Hors d'Oeuvres
New Millennium Soul Food

Mardi Gras Grub (Phat Tuesday)
Valentine's Day Decadence

▪ SPRING ▪

Lara's Cuban Comfort Meal
Ludie and Elizabeth's Afro-Latina Tapas
Simply Macrobiotic

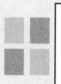

Summer

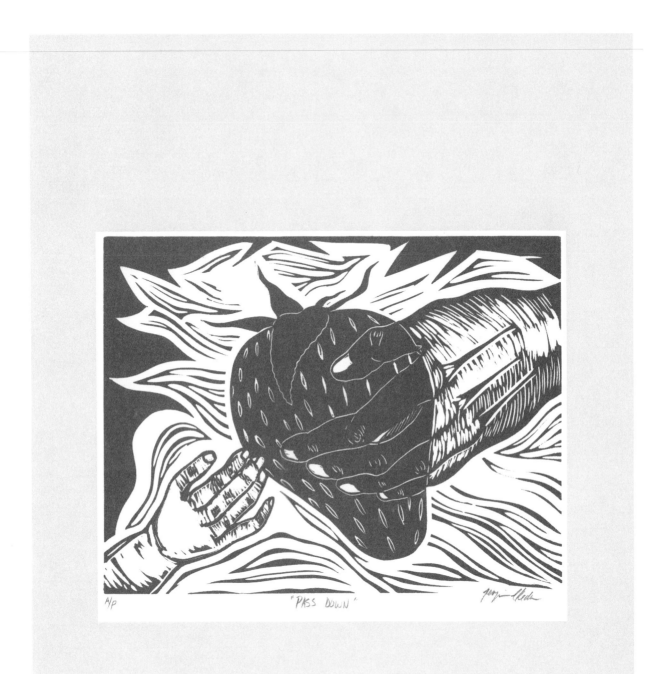

A/P   "PASS DOWN"

DOWN SOUTH OF THE U.S. BORDER
(LA LINEA)

■ ■ ■

Corn on the Cob with Tabasco Butter

■

*Fish Tacos with Cherry Tomato–Rosemary Salsa and
Spicy All-Green Guacamole*

■

Black Beans and Brown Rice

■

Fresh Pineapple, Jicama, and Mint Salad

■ ■ ■

Soundtrack
(provided by Lila Downs)

Elliot Goldenthal, *Soundtrack from the movie* Frida
Mono Blanco y Stone Lips, *El Mundo Se Va a Acabar*
Lucha Reyes, *Serie Platino*
Son de Madera, *Son de Madera*
Toña la Negra, *La Sensacion Jarocha*

Bonus Soundtrack (Lila Downs's Albums)
Una Sangre (One Blood)
Border (La Linea)
Tree of Life (Yutu Tata Árbol de la Vida)
La Sandunga

■ ■ ■

For our second Grub party, we served a variation of this meal on rustic wooden tables in the lush backyard of a friend's bungalow in the heart of West Berkeley. The Mexican-inspired menu made for a perfect summer evening meal. The recipes were inspired by meals I'd eaten at some of the best taquerias (outside of Mexico, of course) in San Francisco's Mission District. We were able to buy most of the ingredients from local farmers at a farmers' market. We served tortilla chips that were made at a nearby Mexican restaurant, and the dried spices and cheeses came from a neighborhood Mexican grocery store.

WHILE THE FARMER SLEEPS

While the farmer sleeps he hears the faint cries of
The priests who stand at the four corners of his

Field, chanting the ancient prayer
Of forgiveness for cutting the first Ear of Corn

He sees Selu, the Old Corn Woman of the
Cherokees searching for the path through the

Fields to his house at harvest time
He watches Selu come to him in her flayed deerskin dress

He feels her blood drip on his own body, the blood
Of Selu, who was slain by her disobedient children

Who refused to listen when she told them:

You may grow the maize
Our forefathers gave you,

But never, never
Change its soul.

MARC LAPPÉ
from *No Levity in the Morgue*

Corn on the Cob with Tabasco Butter

PREPARATION TIME: 5 minutes
COOKING TIME: 10 minutes

BONUS FILM SUGGESTION: The Future of Food (2004), directed by Deborah Koons Garcia. This film offers an in-depth investigation into the disturbing truth behind genetically engineered foods.

Eating fresh corn on the cob coated with green Tabasco sauce was a trick that my friends Andre and Lara Canty-Swapp shared with me back in 1998. I've been eating it like this ever since. Be careful, because 40 percent of the corn grown in the United States is genetically modified. Purchasing organic corn and corn products is the best way to make sure that you're not eating the genetically modified stuff.

Coarse sea salt
4 ears of corn, broken in half
¼ cup green Tabasco sauce
2 tablespoons melted unsalted butter
Freshly ground black pepper

- In a large pot bring 6 quarts of water to a boil. Add 2 teaspoons salt and bring back to a boil. Remove from the heat and add the corn. Cover and let sit in the hot water for 10 minutes.
- Meanwhile, in a large serving bowl combine the Tabasco sauce, butter, and ¼ teaspoon salt and mix well. Remove the corn from the water using tongs, and add to the bowl. Toss the corn, using the tongs, until it is coated well. Add black pepper to taste.

Having a server at a restaurant grind fresh pepper onto your plate is not just fanfare. As with other spices, freshly ground pepper is a lot more flavorful and aromatic than preground. Buying whole peppercorns and grinding them just before adding to a dish will ensure that you have the strongest flavors. Make sure you add the pepper just at the end of cooking, as it loses its flavor and aroma if cooked for too long. As with other spices, store peppercorns in a tightly sealed dark glass container in a cool, dark, and dry place. Once ground, use pepper within three months.

Fish Tacos with Cherry Tomato–Rosemary Salsa and Spicy All-Green Guacamole

PREPARATION TIME: 30 minutes
INACTIVE PREPARATION TIME: 30 minutes
COOKING TIME: 15 minutes

When I was testing recipes for this book, I "tested" this recipe more than any of the others. There wasn't anything wrong; nothing needed fixing. I just got it so right the first time I couldn't stop eating it.

This salsa is always a big hit. The cherry tomatoes make it sweeter than typical tomato salsas, and most people will spend a few moments trying to figure out what else makes it taste so different. You can keep it a secret, or tell them: it's the rosemary. If you plan to snack on chips before dinner, you can double the salsa recipe and use half of it to accompany them.

SALSA
1 pint cherry tomatoes, stemmed and halved (or quartered if using
large cherry tomatoes) with a serrated knife

½ cup diced red onion (from 1 small onion)

1 garlic clove, minced

1 tablespoon minced fresh rosemary

¼ habanero chile, seeded and finely chopped

1½ tablespoons fresh lemon juice (from about 1 lemon)

½ teaspoon coarse sea salt

2 teaspoons extra-virgin olive oil

Guacamole

2 ripe Hass avocados, peeled and pitted (reserve the pits)

3 tablespoons minced fresh cilantro

3 tablespoons thinly sliced scallions

1 garlic clove, minced

1 jalapeño chile, seeded and finely chopped

1½ tablespoons fresh lime juice

Pinch of cayenne pepper

Coarse sea salt

Fish Tacos

16 corn tortillas, at room temperature

3 to 4 catfish fillets (about 1½ pounds), cut in half horizontally
    and then cut into ¼-inch vertical slices

Coarse sea salt

1½ teaspoons paprika

1 tablespoon extra-virgin olive oil

⅓ cup fresh lemon juice

2 tablespoons chopped fresh cilantro, for garnish

1 cup grated pepper jack cheese (optional)

4 cups romaine lettuce cut into chiffonade (see Box, page 145)

Your favorite hot sauce

FOR THE SALSA

- In a large bowl, combine all the ingredients and stir well. Cover and refrigerate for at least 30 minutes to allow the flavors to combine. Bring just to room temperature before serving.

FOR THE GUACAMOLE

- In a medium bowl, combine the avocado and cilantro and, using the back of a spoon, mash the avocado until creamy but still textured. Add the, scallions, garlic, jalapeño, lime juice, cayenne, and ½ teaspoon salt and mix well. Add the pits, which will prevent rapid browning. Cover and refrigerate while you make the tacos.

FOR THE FISH TACOS

- Prepare a steamer by filling it with ¼ to ½ inch water and bring to a boil. Wrap the tortillas in a kitchen towel, place them in the steamer insert, and cover the steamer. Then reduce the heat to a simmer and steam the tortillas for 2 minutes. Turn off the heat and let them stand, covered, until dinner time, at least 15 minutes, or up to 25 minutes.
- Meanwhile, in a large bowl, combine the fish, 1 teaspoon salt, and the paprika. With clean hands or with clean disposable plastic kitchen gloves, massage the spices into the fish for 2 to 3 minutes. (Massaging the spices into the fish works to thoroughly and evenly season each slice. Just wash your hands well when you're done.)
- Warm a large sauté pan over high heat until hot. Add the olive oil and warm it for 30 seconds, until hot. Add the catfish and sauté for about 1½ minutes, until partially cooked, tossing the fish chunks with a heatproof spatula. Add the lemon juice and cook for 1½ minutes more, or until the fish is cooked through. Remove from the heat. With a slotted spoon, transfer fish slices to a serving bowl and garnish with the cilantro.

TO ASSEMBLE

- Place the cheese, if using, lettuce, salsa, and guacamole in beautiful individual serving bowls. Allow guests to assemble their own tacos, adding hot sauce as desired. I assemble my tacos the following way: stack 2 tortillas; use a slotted spoon to scoop out 2 heaping tablespoons of fish and evenly spread over the top tortilla; add a few dashes of my favorite hot sauce; spread 2 tablespoons of cheese on top of the fish; spread 2 heaping tablespoons of salsa on top of the cheese; add a couple of dollops of guacamole on top of the salsa; and pile lettuce on top.

VARIATIONS

- Black beans can be substituted for the fish.
- If you like crunchy tacos (like me), warm ¾ inch olive oil in a large nonstick frying pan over medium-high heat. Add 2 corn tortillas and fry for about 30 seconds, until crisp, pressing down with a metal spatula to prevent buckling. Transfer to a paper towel–lined plate to drain. Repeat with the remaining tortillas, stacking them as they're fried. Cover with aluminum foil and keep warm in a low oven.

CHIFFONADE

Chiffonade refers to thin strips or shreds of vegetables or herbs, either lightly sautéed or used raw as a garnish. To prepare lettuce chiffonade, first remove the stems and reserve them for a salad. Next, stack four or five leaves on top of one another. Roll them into a tight cylinder and slice crosswise with a sharp knife, cutting the leaves into thin strips. Rinse the leaves in cold water, drain in a colander, and spin dry in a salad spinner.

Black Beans and Brown Rice

PREPARATION TIME: 10 minutes
INACTIVE PREPARATION TIME: Overnight
COOKING TIME: 1 hour

You'll probably have some leftovers. I like to eat mine with scrambled free-range, organic eggs, salsa, and warm tortillas for breakfast the next day.

SOAKING AND COOKING RICE

Soaking

Soaking rice usually shortens cooking time and makes it more digestible. If soaking at room temperature, 30 minutes to 1 hour is sufficient. I usually cover mine and soak it overnight in the refreigerator. I like to cook my rice in the soaking water. You'll need to make sure you add the correct amount of water needed for cooking your rice. Generally, the ratio of rice to water is 1 cup rice to 1½ to 2 cups water. Add your sea salt (¼ to ½ teaspoon) to the water before soaking, too.

Cooking

Add your rice and water to a heavy pot or saucepan. Bring to a boil over high heat, then reduce the heat to medium-low. Simmer for 45 minutes to 1 hour, or until all the liquid is absorbed. Don't lift the lid, as this releases steam and slows down the cooking process. Unless the recipe calls for it, do not stir your rice until it's done. You will disturb the steam holes and make it harder to cook. Always let your rice steam with the lid on for 5 to 10 minutes when done, then fluff with a fork.

BROWN RICE

1 cup short-grain brown rice

Coarse sea salt

BLACK BEANS

1½ cups dried black beans

2-inch strip kombu

Coarse sea salt

2 tablespoons extra-virgin olive oil

1½ medium red onions, diced

1½ medium yellow onions, diced

4 garlic cloves, minced

1 large jalapeño chile, seeded and finely chopped

1 tablespoon ground cumin

2 teaspoons dried oregano

2 tablespoons balsamic vinegar

Freshly ground black pepper

FOR THE BROWN RICE

- In a medium bowl, combine the brown rice, ¼ teaspoon salt, and 2¼ cups water. Swish the rice around, cover, and refrigerate overnight.
- Place the rice and water in a medium saucepan over medium heat. Bring to a boil, then cover, reduce the heat to low, and cook for 50 minutes.
- Remove from heat and steam with cover on for at least 10 minutes, then fluff with a fork before serving.

FOR THE BLACK BEANS

- While the rice is soaking, sort and rinse the black beans. In a large bowl, combine the beans with 6 cups water. Cover and refrigerate overnight. Drain.
- While the rice is cooking, combine the black beans, 6 cups of water, and kombu in a large saucepan and bring to a boil. Skim off any foam, reduce the heat to low, and simmer, partially covered, for 25 minutes.

- Meanwhile, warm the olive oil in a large saucepan over medium heat. Add the red and yellow onions and sauté until softened, about 10 minutes. Add the garlic, jalapeño, cumin, oregano, and 1½ teaspoons salt and cook, stirring constantly, until fragrant, about 3 minutes. Remove the kombu from the beans, add the onion mixture to the beans, and continue simmering until the beans are tender, about another 30 minutes.
- Stir in the vinegar and season with salt and black pepper to taste. Serve the brown rice on individual serving plates and spoon the beans (using a slotted spoon) on top.

Fresh Pineapple, Jicama, and Mint Salad

PREPARATION TIME: 20 minutes

INACTIVE PREPARATION TIME: At least 2 hours, or overnight

I also enjoy this salad with plain yogurt as a light breakfast or snack.

2 cups fresh orange juice (from about 6 oranges)
1 small jicama (about 1½ pounds),
   peeled and cut into ½-inch cubes
2 cups fresh pineapple cut into ½-inch cubes
½ cup chopped fresh mint

- Combine all the ingredients in a large bowl. With clean hands toss well for 2 to 3 minutes until well combined. Cover and refrigerate for at least 2 hours, or overnight. (If letting sit overnight, wait to put the mint in until 30 minutes before serving.)
- Transfer to a serving bowl and serve with a slotted spoon.

Food for Thought

Be mindful of the Mexican and other immigrant agricultural workers who cross the border and toil in our fields to provide the United States with a bountiful food supply.

▮ TIPS FOR PREPARING THIS MENU ▮

- Soak the rice and the black beans overnight before cooking them. If possible, cook the black beans the day before: they'll be even more flavorful.
- Make the salad the night before (but hold the mint until 30 minutes before serving).
- Make the salsa a few hours before guests arrive.
- If you're not drinking the recommended wine, a good Mexican beer goes well with this menu.
- Prepare all the guacamole ingredients except for the avocados in advance and make the guacamole at the table right before the meal starts.

ITAL GRUB

■ ■ ■

Sun-Kissed Fruit, Avocado, and Romaine Salad with
Citrus-Ginger Vinaigrette

■

Red Bell Peppers Stuffed with Seitan,
Roasted Tomatoes, and Rice

■

Likkle Chile–Roasted Plantains

■

Not-Too-Sweet Sorrel

■ ■ ■

Soundtrack
(provided by Laurent "Tippy" Alfred)

Burning Spear, *Marcus Garvey*
Hugh Mundell, *Africa Must Be Free By 1983*
Midnite, *Unpolished*
Sizzla, *Black Woman & Child*
Bob Marley and the Wailers, *Catch a Fire*

■ ■ ■

When I first moved to New York in 1997, I lived in a predominately West Indian neighborhood in Brooklyn. I had no problem maintaining my meat-free diet, as there was a Rastafarian-owned health food store or vegetarian restaurant on almost every corner. I spent 'nuff money on crispy veggie patties, spicy rice and peas, fried sweet plantains, hearty vegetable roti, tart sorrel, spicy ginger beer, and Ital stew. Memories of my year in Crown Heights inspired this menu.

"Ital" is taken from the word vital, with the revolutionary use of "I"—which is employed throughout Rastafari jargon as a way to emphasize the oneness and unity of life. The term means a natural and healthy way of life. Ital food promotes a healthy mind, body, spirit, and environment. Ital food is as fresh as possible, free from additives, preservatives, and other chemicals, and in most cases dairy free.

Ital food usually does not contain added salt, as many Rastafarians see salt as unnatural. Since it helps draw out the essential flavors in food, avoiding added salt in this menu forced me to be extra creative with herbs, spices, and cooking techniques. These recipes are clearly Caribbean-inspired, but any food can be Ital if it is prepared in accordance with Rasta principles.

Sun-Kissed Fruit, Avocado, and Romaine Salad with Citrus-Ginger Vinaigrette

PREPARATION TIME: 15 minutes

Edible sunshine.

VINAIGRETTE
2 tablespoons fresh orange juice
1 tablespoon fresh lemon juice
1 tablespoon fresh ginger juice (see Box, page 152)
½ teaspoon Dijon mustard
7 tablespoons extra-virgin olive oil
Freshly ground black pepper

SALAD
2 ripe mangoes, peeled, pitted, and cubed
1 jalapeño chile, seeded and finely chopped
½ cup fresh orange juice
2 large Hass avocados, peeled, pitted, and cubed

1 teaspoon fresh lemon juice

½ teaspoon paprika

1 large head romaine lettuce, chopped into bite-size pieces

½ cup golden raisins

Freshly ground white pepper

FOR THE VINAIGRETTE

- In a small bowl, whisk together the orange juice, lemon juice, ginger juice, and mustard. Slowly whisk in the olive oil. Add black pepper to taste.

FOR THE SALAD

- In a small bowl, combine the mangoes and jalapeño with the orange juice and set aside for 10 minutes, tossing every few minutes. Drain.
- In a small bowl combine the avocados with the lemon juice. Gently toss together. Sprinkle with the paprika.
- In a large bowl, toss the lettuce with enough vinaigrette to coat well.
- To serve, divide the salad among 4 plates in the following way: pile a quarter of the lettuce on 1 side of the plate, a quarter of the mango mixture in the middle of the plate, and a quarter of the avocados on the other side of the plate. Sprinkle 2 tablespoons raisins and white pepper to taste over each plate.

JUICING GINGER

The easiest way to get juice from ginger is to feed it into an electric juicer and let technology do all the work. But if you don't have a juicer, here's another way: First, grate your ginger knobs on a fine grater (don't worry about peeling them). If you're in a hurry you can pulverize them in a food processor to get pulp. Next, wrap the pulp in cheesecloth and squeeze to extract all the juice. You can also squeeze the pulp through your hands without the cheesecloth, in batches, and then strain the juice.

Red Bell Peppers Stuffed with Seitan, Roasted Tomatoes, and Rice

■ ■ ■

PREPARATION TIME: 1 hour
INACTIVE PREPARATION TIME: Overnight
COOKING TIME: 1 hour and 25 minutes

My inspiration for this recipe came from my mom's stuffed green bell peppers. I like to use red bell peppers because they are riper, sweeter, and more nutritious than green.

This recipe is written for 4 servings but there is enough filling to serve 5. So if you're expecting an extra guest, simply have an extra bell pepper on hand.

1 cup brown basmati rice

3 tablespoons extra-virgin olive oil

8 plum tomatoes

6 garlic cloves, unpeeled

4 large red bell peppers,
*   tops cut off and seeded*

½ cup finely diced yellow onion

½ cup finely diced red onion

½ cup finely diced green bell pepper

1 pound seitan, finely chopped (see Note, page 155)

½ teaspoon ground allspice

½ teaspoon ground cumin

½ teaspoon freshly ground black pepper

¼ teaspoon red pepper flakes

⅛ teaspoon cayenne pepper

1 garlic clove, minced

1 tablespoon apple cider vinegar

¼ cup chopped fresh thyme,
*   plus 4 or 5 sprigs for garnish*

- In a medium bowl, combine the rice and 2 cups water. Cover and refrigerate overnight. Drain.
- Preheat the broiler.
- Warm a medium saucepan over medium heat. Add the rice and cook for about 4 minutes, until the water has evaporated and the rice smells nutty, stirring often with a wooden spoon. Add 1 tablespoon of the olive oil and sauté for 1 additional minute. Add 2 cups water and bring to a boil. Cover, reduce the heat to low, and cook for 45 minutes, or until the rice is tender and all the water has been absorbed. Remove from the heat, let stand with the lid on for 10 minutes, then fluff with a fork. Remove the lid and set aside to cool a bit.
- While the rice is cooking, line a baking sheet with parchment paper. Place the tomatoes on the baking sheet, and place the unpeeled garlic cloves in a corner of the baking sheet. Broil fairly close to the heat source until the tomatoes and garlic cloves begin to blacken, about 10 minutes. Remove the baking sheet from the oven and transfer the garlic to a small bowl to cool. Turn the tomatoes with tongs and return them to the broiler. Continue to broil until the tomatoes begin to blacken on the other side, about 10 more minutes. Remove from the oven and set aside to cool. Reduce the oven temperature to 350°F.
- When cooled, slip the garlic cloves out of their skins and transfer to the bowl of a food processor and process until smooth. Add the tomatoes and their juices from the baking sheet. Process in 2 or 3 quick pulses; the mixture should be chunky. Transfer to a bowl and set aside.
- Bring 5 quarts of water to a boil in a large pot over high heat. Add the red bell peppers, in 2 batches if necessary, and blanch for 1 minute, or until just slightly softened. Make sure the bell peppers stay immersed in the water, pushing them down with a spider if necessary. Remove with a spider or slotted spoon and set aside upside down in a colander to drain.
- Warm the remaining 2 tablespoons olive oil in a large sauté pan or skillet over medium heat. Add the yellow and red onions and diced green bell peppers and sauté for 5 minutes, or until softened. Add the seitan, allspice, cumin, black pepper, red pepper flakes, and cayenne and sauté, stirring frequently, for 3 minutes, or until the seitan starts to brown. Add the minced garlic and sauté for about 2 minutes, until the garlic has softened. Remove from the heat, add the rice, 2 cups of

the tomato-garlic mixture (reserve the rest for topping the finished peppers), the vinegar, and thyme and stir well.

- Stuff the bell peppers with the rice mixture and transfer them to a baking dish large enough to fit the bell peppers snugly. Loosely cover with aluminum foil and bake for 30 minutes, or until the peppers are tender.
- Remove from oven and top the bell peppers with the remaining tomato-garlic mixture. Cool to room temperature before serving (if it's a hot summer day), or serve hot, garnished with a sprig of thyme.

Note: Store-bought seitan usually contains salt.

Likkle Chile–Roasted Plantains

PREPARATION TIME: 5 minutes
COOKING TIME: 30 minutes

Bonus Film Suggestion: Life and Debt (2001), directed by Stephanie Black. This documentary brilliantly explores the ways international financial institutions such as the International Monetary Fund and the World Bank have had an impact on the Jamaican economy over the past twenty-five years. It is a powerful story of the devastation of a particular type of globalization.

Likkle = little in West Indian patois. Roasting ripe plantains intensifies their sweetness. The red chile adds some color and spiciness.

4 large very ripe yellow plantains
3 tablespoons extra-virgin olive oil
½ to 1 habanero chile, seeded and minced (see Note)

- Preheat the oven to 375°F. Lightly oil a baking dish, or line it with parchment paper.
- Cut off the ends of the plantains. Cut a slit down the length of each plantain skin and remove the skin. Cut each plantain diagonally into ¼-inch pieces.

- In a large bowl, combine the plantains with the olive oil and toss well. Add the habanero and toss again.
- Transfer the plantains to the prepared baking dish and roast for about 30 minutes, gently tossing or shaking the plantains around every 10 minutes, until tender and lightly browned.
- Serve hot or cool to room temperature before serving.

Note: It's a good idea to wear rubber gloves when handling habanero chiles, especially if you have sensitive skin.

NOT-SO-OBVIOUS KITCHEN GEAR #2: PARCHMENT PAPER

Using parchment paper usually decreases the amount of fat needed for cooking, and it is great for preventing food from sticking to baking sheets and roasting pans. Using parchment paper will also extend the life of your baking sheets and roasting pans.

Not-Too-Sweet Sorrel

PREPARATION TIME: 5 minutes
INACTIVE PREPARATION TIME: 2 hours
COOKING TIME: 20 minutes
YIELD: about half a gallon

Sorrel is a traditional Caribbean drink made from dried *Hibiscus sabdariffa*, commonly referred to as Jamaican or red sorrel. This sorrel should not be mistaken for garden sorrel (*Rumex acetosa*). You can buy dried sorrel in Caribbean and African specialty stores. Ask for dried hibiscus flowers if shopping elsewhere.

1 cup (about 1 ounce) dried red sorrel

½ cup coarsely grated fresh ginger

½ cup organic raw cane sugar

- Combine 8 cups of water, the sorrel, and ginger in a large saucepan over high heat. Bring to a boil, then reduce the heat and simmer for 20 minutes. Remove from heat.
- Meanwhile, make a simple syrup by combining 1 cup of water with the sugar in a small saucepan placed over low heat. Stir well until hot to the touch and the sugar is completely dissolved. Add to the sorrel drink, stir well, and let stand, covered, for 2 hours.
- Strain into a pitcher and refrigerate until cold.
- Serve over ice.

Food for Thought

Economic globalization has resulted in the decline of the banana and sugar industries in most Caribbean countries.

▪ TIPS FOR PREPARING THIS MENU ▪

- Soak the rice in the refrigerator the night before.
- Make the sorrel the day before and refrigerate it.
- Make the vinaigrette for the salad a few hours before serving and keep it refrigerated.
- Make the filling for the peppers and blanch the peppers 1 hour before stuffing them.
- Serve the salad as a first course, followed by the stuffed peppers on a plate surrounded by roasted plantains, along with tall slender glasses of ice-cold sorrel.

Beets, Limes, and Rice:
Salad Selection for Heads

■ ■ ■

Balsamic-Roasted Beetnuts Salad

■

Cucumberslice, Mint, and Lime Salad

■

Wild-Style Salad

■ ■ ■

Soundtrack

(provided by Bobbito Garcia, a.k.a. DJ Cucumberslice)

Bobbito, *Earthtones*

DJ Spinna and Bobbito, *The Wonder of Stevie*

Organized Konfusion, *Organized Konfusion*

Syreeta, *Syreeta*

■ ■ ■

SUMMER '74

black/brown bodies—breathe
billows of beats and lyrics
then sink into peace

BRYANT TERRY

Balsamic Roasted Beetnuts Salad

PREPARATION TIME: 50 minutes
INACTIVE PREPARATION TIME: At least 4 hours, or up to overnight
COOKING TIME: 50 minutes

BONUS SOUNDTRACK SUGGESTION: The Beatnuts, *Street Level.* This is the first full-length project of the Beatnuts, a highly respected rapper/producer team.

My friend Marla Teyolia suggested that I use nut "cheese" for this salad instead of goat cheese, which I had planned to use, since she does not eat dairy products. I did, and nut cheese works perfectly, as it balances the sweet beets and pecans.

NUT CHEESE

1 cup sunflower seeds
½ cup pine nuts
1 garlic clove, minced
2 tablespoons minced fresh basil
1 tablespoon fresh lemon juice
1 tablespoon apple cider vinegar
2 teaspoons extra-virgin olive oil
2 teaspoons tamari

SALAD

4 medium beets, scrubbed and tops trimmed but root tails intact
Coarse sea salt
½ cup pecan halves
½ cup plus 4 teaspoons extra-virgin olive oil
2 teaspoons organic raw cane sugar
2 tablespoons pure maple syrup
2 tablespoons red balsamic vinegar

2 tablespoons white balsamic vinegar or apple cider vinegar

1 teaspoon Dijon mustard

Freshly ground black pepper

FOR THE NUT CHEESE

- In a large bowl combine the sunflower seeds and pine nuts and add water to cover. Cover and soak in the refrigerator for at least 4 hours, or up to overnight. Drain.
- Preheat the oven to 375°F. Line a baking pan with parchment paper.
- Transfer the sunflower seeds and pine nuts to a blender. Add water to cover and blend until creamy, adding more water if necessary.
- In batches, pour a cup of the nut mixture into the middle of a piece of cheesecloth or a clean kitchen towel. Squeeze out all the liquid and place the remaining "cheese" into a small bowl. Add the garlic, basil, lemon juice, vinegar, olive oil, and tamari and mix well.
- Spread the mixture ½ inch thick over the prepared baking pan and bake until lightly browned, about 10 minutes. Remove from the oven and set aside to cool. Leave the oven on. Spoon up 16 heaping teaspoons of the nut cheese and shape each teaspoon into small balls with your hands. Set aside.

FOR THE SALAD

- Lower the oven temperature to 275°F.
- Combine the beets, 3 quarts cold water, and 1 teaspoon salt in a medium pot over high heat. Bring to a boil and boil uncovered for 20 to 30 minutes, or until the beets are easily pierced with a knife. Drain. Peel the beets by holding them under cold running water and rubbing their skins off with your fingers or a clean towel.
- Meanwhile, spread the pecans on a large baking sheet and toast for 5 minutes.
- Warm 1 tablespoon of the olive oil in a small skillet over medium heat. Add the pecans, sugar, and maple syrup and cook, stirring constantly, until the pecans are thoroughly coated with the syrup, about 4 minutes.
- Transfer the nuts to parchment paper to cool, then coarsely chop the nuts.
- Increase the oven temperature to 400°F.
- Trim the tails off of the bottom of the beets and reserve them for the vinaigrette. Cut the beets into quarters. In a medium bowl, toss the beets with 4 teaspoons of

the olive oil. Place cut side up on a baking sheet and roast for 15 minutes. Remove the beets from the oven, place them back in the bowl, and toss in the red balsamic vinegar. Return cut side up to the baking sheet and cook for an additional 5 minutes, or until they are slightly crisp on the edges. Set the beets aside to cool.

- In a blender, combine the reserved beet tails with the white balsamic vinegar, mustard, ½ teaspoon salt, and black pepper to taste. Blend while slowly pouring in the remaining 7 tablespoons olive oil.
- Place 4 beet wedges on each plate and drizzle with the vinaigrette. Place 4 nut cheese balls on each plate. Divide the pecans among the plates.

NOT-SO-OBVIOUS KITCHEN GEAR #3: CHEESECLOTH

Cheesecloth is great for straining broths and other liquids, squeezing seedless juice from citrus fruits, extracting juice from grated ginger pulp, making nut milks, and more.

Cucumberslice, Mint, and Lime Salad

PREPARATION TIME: 45 minutes

INACTIVE PREPARATION TIME: At least 30 minutes, or up to 2 hours.

BONUS SOUNDTRACK SUGGESTION: MF DOOM, *Operation Doomsday.* This album, an instant hip-hop cult classic, was the first full-length album released by MF DOOM (formerly Zev Love X of KMD). Bobbito Garcia (DJ Cucumberslice) was the executive producer and a featured vocalist.

This is a great summer salad, as cucumbers and mint are both cooling foods. It was inspired by a salad I prepared with my friend and mentor Stefanie Bryn Sacks, an amazing culinary nutritionist.

3 medium cucumbers, peeled and thinly sliced

¼ cup fresh lime juice

⅓ cup chopped fresh mint

Coarse sea salt

Freshly ground white pepper

- In a large bowl, combine the cucumbers, lime juice, and mint. With clean hands, toss well for 1 minute. Add ½ teaspoon salt and white pepper to taste. Toss for an additional minute. Cover and refrigerate for at least 30 minutes, or up to 2 hours. Taste and add more salt and pepper if needed.

Wild-Style Salad

PREPARATION TIME: 20 minutes

INACTIVE PREPARATION TIME: Overnight, plus 1 hour and 30 minutes

COOKING TIME: 45 minutes

Bonus Film Suggestion: Wild Style (1982), directed by Charlie Ahearn. This is a classic hip-hop film that captures the culture at its birth in the Bronx.

Salad

1 cup wild rice, rinsed and soaked overnight in the refrigerator

Coarse sea salt

1 red bell pepper, seeded and diced

¼ cup diced carrots

½ cup thinly sliced celery

½ cup golden raisins

½ cup thinly sliced scallions

½ cup cashews, toasted and chopped

DRESSING

3 tablespoons apple cider vinegar

1 tablespoon fresh lemon juice

2 teaspoons Dijon mustard

1 teaspoon pure maple syrup

1 garlic clove, minced

2 tablespoons chopped parsley

Fine sea salt

Freshly ground white pepper

¼ cup extra-virgin olive oil

FOR THE SALAD

- Combine the wild rice with 3 cups of water in a medium saucepan over high heat. Bring to a boil, add ½ teaspoon salt, reduce the heat to low, cover, and simmer for 30 minutes, or until all the water is absorbed.

- Remove from the heat, transfer to a strainer or sieve, and rinse under cold water until the rice is completely cooled.

- In a large bowl, combine the cooked rice, bell pepper, carrots, celery, raisins, scallions, and cashews with clean hands.

FOR THE DRESSING

- In a small mixing bowl, combine the vinegar, lemon juice, mustard, maple syrup, garlic, parsley, ½ teaspoon salt, and white pepper to taste. Mix well. Slowly pour in the olive oil, whisking until emulsified.

- Pour the dressing over the rice and toss well with clean hands. Cover and refrigerate for 1 hour to allow flavors to combine.

- Remove the rice from the refrigerator 30 minutes before serving.

Food for Thought

As Dead Prez says, it's bigger than hip-hop, hip-hop, hip-hop . . .

TIPS FOR PREPARING THIS MENU

- Toast and chop the pecans the day before.
- Make the nut cheese the day before, but do not bake it until a few hours before serving the salad.
- Soak the wild rice in the refrigerator overnight.
- Make the dressing for the Wild-Style Salad the night before.

AFRODIASPORIC COOKOUT

■ ■ ■

Grilled Corn and Heirloom Tomato Salad
with Fresh Basil

■

Shrimp and Veggie Kabobs with
Mixed Herb Marinade

■

Fresh Green Beans with Garlicky Citrus Vinaigrette

■

Good Grilled Okra

■

Ginger Beer

■ ■ ■

Soundtrack
(provided by Robin D. G. Kelley)

Burnt Sugar, *Black Sex Y'all Liberation & Random Bloody Violets*
The Marvin Sewell Group, *The Worker's Dance*
Jason Moran, *Same Mother*
Mutabaruka, *Any Which Way . . . Freedom*
Randy Weston, *Uhuru Afrika/Highlife: Music of the New African Nations*

■ ■ ■

Read with a whiny voice: "It's too slimy!" That's the usual response from folks when I ask if they like okra. Don't get me wrong—the way most people cook okra leaves it pitifully limp and glue-like. But my friend Holly Roberson recently turned me on to a way to prepare it that will convert even die-hard okra haters—grilling. Holly swore I would love newly picked okra coated with a light mixture of fresh squeezed lemon juice, extra-virgin olive oil, and coarse sea salt and then grilled until crisp.

Now I have had okra prepared in every way imaginable: my maternal grandmother used to pickle it for the winter; my mom would sauté it along with corn and juicy tomatoes from our garden; and when I lived in New Orleans I always ate it in seafood gumbo, where it is used as a thickener. But grilling is, by far, the best way that I've ever had okra. This whole meal was inspired by those crisp purple "lady fingers" on skewers. (Yes, there is purple okra!)

Since okra is a native African plant (historians believe it originated over 10,000 years ago in what is now Ethiopia) and is used in African, Afro-Caribbean, and African-American cuisine, I created recipes for this menu that draw inspiration from dishes that I've eaten from different parts of the African Diaspora. Enjoy this meal at an afternoon cookout with family and friends.

Grilled Corn and Heirloom Tomato Salad with Fresh Basil

PREPARATION TIME: 10 minutes
INACTIVE PREPARATION TIME: 1 hour
COOKING TIME: 20 to 25 minutes

This dish is inspired by "Okra, Corn, and Tomatoes," a Southern classic. In August heirloom tomatoes are at their peak, and you can easily find them at farmers' markets. Some health food stores and conventional grocery stores carry them as well.

4 ears of corn, silks removed, husks left on, and soaked in cold salted
  water for 1 hour
1¾ pounds heirloom tomatoes of varying shapes, sizes, and colors
16 basil leaves (preferably purple), each leaf torn into a few pieces
Best-quality extra-virgin olive oil
Coarse sea salt
Freshly ground black pepper

- Preheat the grill or broiler. Remove the corn from the soaking water. If grilling, place the corn on the grill. Close the cover and grill, turning frequently with tongs, until cooked thoroughly, 20 to 25 minutes. Remove the corn from the grill and let cool.
- If broiling, place the corn about 6 inches from the heat for 20 to 25 minutes, turning occasionally, until cooked thoroughly. Let cool.
- Remove the husks and cut the kernels off the corn cobs. Place in a bowl and set aside.
- Cut the tomatoes in various styles to enhance presentation—halves, quarters, and slices.
- Divide the corn and tomatoes evenly among 4 plates. Divide the basil evenly on top, drizzle with olive oil, and sprinkle with salt and black pepper.

Shrimp and Veggie Kabobs with Mixed Herb Marinade

PREPARATION TIME: 20 minutes
INACTIVE PREPARATION TIME: At least 3 hours, or overnight
COOKING TIME: 15 minutes

Kabobs are the quintessential cookout food. Here's to you, Dad.

MARINADE
¼ cup fresh lemon juice
¾ cup fresh orange juice
¾ cup fresh lime juice
½ cup apple juice
2 tablespoons minced fresh basil
2 tablespoons minced fresh parsley
2 tablespoons minced fresh rosemary

2 garlic cloves, minced

2 serrano chiles, seeded and minced

1½ teaspoons coarse sea salt

½ cup extra-virgin olive oil

KABOBS

Sixteen 12-inch wooden skewers, soaked in water for at least 30 minutes

32 large shrimp (about 1 pound), peeled and deveined (see Note)

24 cremini mushrooms, stemmed and cleaned

1 large red bell pepper, cored, seeded, and cut into 1-inch squares

1 large orange bell pepper, cored, seeded, and cut into 1-inch squares

1 large yellow bell pepper, cored, seeded, and cut into 1-inch squares

1 large onion, cut into 4 vertical pieces and then halved

- In a large bowl combine all the marinade ingredients and whisk well.
- Add all the vegetables and the shrimp to the marinade, cover, and refrigerate for at least 3 hours or overnight, stirring occasionally.
- Preheat the grill or broiler.
- Thread the shrimp and vegetables onto the skewers, use 2 wooden skewers per kabob to keep all the ingredients in place. Each kabob should have 4 shrimp, 3 mushrooms, about 2 pieces of each pepper, and several pieces of onion.
- If grilling, place the kabobs on the grill and cook for 4 to 6 minutes on one side, until vegetables start to char. Using a pastry brush, generously apply the marinade to all sides of the kabobs, and then flip over with tongs and cook another 4 to 6 minutes, until the shrimp are just cooked through and the vegetables are slightly charred.
- If broiling, place the kabobs on a foil-lined broiler pan about 6 inches from the heat for 4 to 6 minutes, until vegetables start to char. Using a pastry brush, generously apply the marinade to all sides of the kabobs, and then flip over and cook another 4 to 6 minutes, until the shrimp are just cooked through and the vegetables are slightly charred.

Note: You can substitute 1 to 1½ pounds of finfish cut into ½-inch cubes or 1½ pounds of firm tofu, pressed and cut into ½-inch squares, for the shrimp.

Fresh Green Beans with Garlicky Citrus Vinaigrette

PREPARATION TIME: As long as it takes you to snap the green beans and 5 minutes for the vinaigrette.

COOKING TIME: 5 minutes

Making this dish takes me back to my childhood. My paternal grandfather would make the grandkids harvest buckets of green beans from his garden and snap them on the back porch.

The first time I made this, a friend commented, "The green beans are good because they don't *taste* like green beans!" She probably meant that green beans are usually cooked to death (and depleted of their vital nutrients—vitamin A, B-complex vitamins, calcium, and potassium). With this dish, I blanch them in salted water for a few minutes to take off the edge and brighten the color. The vinaigrette is super-tangy, but it mellows out once the beans are tossed in it.

Coarse sea salt
2 pounds fresh green beans, snapped at each end
2 tablespoons fresh lemon juice
2 tablespoons fresh lime juice
2 tablespoons red wine vinegar
2 teaspoons Dijon mustard

1 tablespoon pure maple syrup

2 large garlic cloves, chopped

1 tablespoon fresh thyme

½ cup extra-virgin olive oil

Freshly ground black pepper

- Bring a large pot of salted water to a boil. Add the green beans and cook 4 to 5 minutes, until tender but still al dente. Drain the green beans into a colander, and shock in a bowl filled with ice water to stop the cooking. Drain again and place in a serving bowl.
- In a blender, combine the lemon and lime juice, vinegar, mustard, maple syrup, garlic, thyme, and ¾ teaspoon salt. Slowly pour in the olive oil with the blender going. Add black pepper to taste.
- Toss the green beans with the vinaigrette.

Good Grilled Okra

PREPARATION TIME: 10 minutes

COOKING TIME: 10 minutes

A great way to eat okra, trust me. Select smaller pods, as they're more tender and less slimy. Refrigerate okra and use it within a few days.

Eighteen 12-inch wooden skewers, soaked in water for at least 30 minutes

1 pound small to medium okra pods

2 teaspoons fresh lemon juice

2 tablespoons extra-virgin olive oil

Coarse sea salt

¼ teaspoon cayenne pepper

½ teaspoon freshly ground black pepper

- Preheat the grill or broiler.
- Wash the okra under cold running water and dry with paper towels.
- In a large bowl, combine the lemon juice, olive oil, 1 teaspoon salt, the cayenne, and black pepper and whisk well.
- Add the okra to the marinade and toss to coat. Thread 5 to 7 okra pods onto 2 skewers each (to keep the okra in place).
- If grilling, place the kabobs on the grill and cook until browned and slightly crisp, 3 to 4 minutes per side, turning with tongs frequently.
- If broiling, place the kabobs about 3 inches from the heat and broil until browned and slightly crisp, 3 to 4 minutes per side, turning with tongs frequently.

Ginger Beer

PREPARATION TIME: 15 minutes

YIELD: About ½ gallon

If you want a sweet, spicy, and refreshing nonalcoholic beverage that increases blood circulation and promotes digestion, this is your drink. Ginger drinks are served in many Caribbean and West African restaurants (along with sorrel). Unfortunately, most restaurants use white sugar as a sweetener. Others, in an attempt to make their drinks healthier, use brown sugar, but contrary to popular belief, brown sugar is not necessarily healthier than white sugar (it's usually just white sugar with a little molasses added to it). In this recipe I use organic raw cane sugar.

½ cup organic raw cane sugar
½ cup fresh ginger juice (from about 2 packed cups
*   freshly grated ginger) (see page 152)*
Zest of 1 lemon
⅓ cup fresh lemon juice (from 3 to 4 lemons)
6 cups sparkling water
Ice

Several fresh mint sprigs, for garnish
Lemon slices, for garnish

- Make a simple syrup by combining ½ cup water with the sugar in a small saucepan over low heat. Stir well until hot to the touch and the sugar is completely dissolved.
- Pour the ginger juice into a pitcher and add the simple syrup, lemon zest, and lemon juice and stir well. Slowly add the sparkling water. Stir well.
- Add the ice. Stir well again. Garnish with the mint sprigs and lemon slices.

Food for Thought

Consider how African cuisine has traveled to the "New World" and shifted the way that we eat.

TIPS FOR PREPARING THIS MENU

- Marinate the shrimp and veggies overnight. They will be really flavorful at grilling time.
- Start soaking the wooden skewers while you heat up the grill.
- Grill the corn first, followed by the shrimp and veggie kabobs. Save the okra kabobs for last.
- The day before, make the ginger beer. Add ice and garnishes just before serving.
- Serve each guest a plate of Grilled Corn and Heirloom Tomato Salad and set up an outdoor buffet with the rest of the dishes.

Straight-Edge Punk Brunch Buffet (DIY)

■ ■ ■

Spicy Tempeh Sausage Patties with
Roasted Yellow Pepper Sauce

■

French Toast with Blueberry Coulis and Fresh Fruit

■

Potato Pancakes

■

Sunflower Sprouts and Baby Mixed Greens Salad
with Yogurt Dressing

■

Stone Fruit Salad

■

Straight-Edge Tangerine Mimosa

■ ■ ■

Soundtrack

(provided by James Spooner)

FIVE MUST-HAVE PUNK ALBUMS	FIVE MUST-HAVE "AFRO-PUNK" ALBUMS
Bad Brains, *Bad Brains*	Bad Brains, *Bad Brains*
Black Flag, *Everything Went Black*	D-FE, *Kemite* (EP)
Minor Threat, *Minor Threat*	Fishbone, *Party at Ground Zero*
Misfits, *Evilive*	X-Ray Specs, *Germ Free Adolescents*
Operation Ivy, *Energy*	Yaphet Kotto, *Government Blankets*

When I was growing up, I was an East Coast hip-hop head, which was pretty out of the ordinary in Memphis during the '80s. So even though I was never a part of the punk scene, I felt a certain kinship to Memphis punks, who were *really* seen as weirdos. I've always been drawn to certain aspects of punk subculture, particularly its "do it yourself" ethic and the straight-edge punk philosophy.

Straight-edge, which evolved out of the punk scene, encourages the avoidance of alcohol, drugs, and casual sex. Many straight-edge punks contribute to political and environmental movements and maintain a vegan diet and lifestyle. Back in the day, I would always run across punk 'zines that included funky vegan recipes. The memory of them inspired this menu. Whether you and your friends are craving sweet, savory, or both, there's something to please everyone in this spread.

Spicy Tempeh Sausage Patties with Roasted Yellow Pepper Sauce

PREPARATION TIME: 10 minutes
INACTIVE PREPARATION TIME: 30 minutes
COOKING TIME: 1 hour

ROASTED YELLOW PEPPER SAUCE

2 yellow bell peppers, roasted, seeded, and chopped
(see Box, page 176)
1 tablespoon extra-virgin olive oil
1 teaspoon fresh lemon juice
Coarse sea salt
Freshly ground black pepper

Tempeh sausages

½ pound (one 8-ounce package) tempeh, cubed

3 cups vegetable stock

Coarse sea salt

2 teaspoons extra-virgin olive oil

1 cup diced yellow onion

½ teaspoon red pepper flakes

⅛ teaspoon cayenne pepper

Freshly ground black pepper

2 garlic cloves, minced

2 teaspoons minced fresh thyme

2 teaspoons minced fresh rosemary

For the roasted yellow pepper sauce

- In a blender or food processor combine the roasted bell peppers, olive oil, lemon juice, 2 tablespoons water, 1 teaspoon salt, and ⅛ teaspoon black pepper. Puree until smooth, adding a little water if necessary. The sauce should pour smoothly but shouldn't be runny. Set aside.

For the tempeh sausages

- Combine the tempeh cubes with the vegetable stock and 1 teaspoon salt in a medium saucepan over medium heat. Bring to a boil, lower the heat, and simmer for 25 minutes, or until the tempeh is moist and saturated with vegetable broth. Remove from the heat and drain the tempeh into a colander.
- Meanwhile, warm the olive oil in a medium sauté pan over medium heat. Add the onion, red pepper flakes, cayenne, ½ teaspoon salt, and ⅛ teaspoon black pepper. Cook for about 7 minutes, until softened, stirring occasionally Add the garlic and cook for 2 more minutes, or until the garlic has softened.

- In a food processor fitted with a metal blade, combine the tempeh cubes with the onion mixture, 1 teaspoon of the thyme, and 1 teaspoon of the rosemary. Pulse until the mixture is smooth and creamy, stopping to scrape the sides as necessary. Scrape the mixture into a bowl, cover, and refrigerate for 30 minutes.
- Preheat the oven to 350°F just before removing the batter from the refrigerator. Lightly oil a baking sheet.
- Form the mixture into 16 walnut-sized balls and flatten them into patties with the palms of your hands. Place the patties on the baking sheet ½ inch apart. Bake for 20 minutes, turning after 10 minutes, until golden brown on each side.
- Warm the yellow pepper sauce in a medium saucepan over medium heat and serve each patty with a dollop of the sauce. Garnish with the remaining teaspoon of thyme and rosemary.

ROASTING PEPPERS

There are a few ways to roast whole peppers: on the top of a gas stove, under a broiler, or on a grill.

If roasting peppers on the burner of a gas stove, place them directly on a low flame and turn frequently with tongs. Remove from the burner when most of the skin is blistered and blackened, then place in a bowl and cover. Let the peppers cool for about 15 minutes, or until you can handle them without burning your hands. Remove from the bowl and peel off the skin with your hands (do not wash the peppers). Cut off the stem end, remove the core and seeds, and cut into strips, or as directed in the recipe. Place in a bowl, toss with olive oil, and refrigerate until ready to use.

If broiling, place the peppers directly on the oven rack and roast until blistered and blackened, about 5 to 7 minutes, turning a few times with tongs. Proceed as above.

If grilling, place the peppers directly on the grill, turning frequently with tongs. Remove when most of the skin is blistered and blackened. Proceed as above.

French Toast with Blueberry Coulis and Fresh Fruit

■ ■ ■

PREPARATION TIME: 15 minutes
COOKING TIME: 50 minutes

This is a sweet and crunchy treat that can be enjoyed as a meal in itself.

COULIS

2 cups fresh blueberries

¼ cup pure maple syrup

1 tablespoon fresh lemon juice

1 teaspoon lemon zest

FRENCH TOAST

8 slices seven-grain bread

2 ripe bananas, sliced

¾ cup rice milk

2 tablespoons almond butter

2 tablespoons pure maple syrup

2 teaspoons pure vanilla extract

½ teaspoon ground cinnamon

¼ freshly grated nutmeg

Fine sea salt

2 teaspoons extra-virgin olive oil, plus more as needed

½ cup fresh blueberries, for garnish

1 cup sliced fresh strawberries, for garnish

½ cup toasted almonds, chopped

FOR THE COULIS

- Combine the blueberries, maple syrup, ¾ cup water, and the lemon juice and zest in a small saucepan over medium heat. Bring to a simmer and simmer until the blueberries are softened and the liquid has thickened, about 10 minutes. Cool for 5 minutes, then puree in a blender in 2 batches. Strain through a fine sieve or cheesecloth, transfer to a bowl, and refrigerate, covered, until completely chilled, at least 30 minutes, while you make the French toast.

For the French toast

- Preheat the oven to 250°F.
- Place the bread slices on a baking sheet and toast them for 20 minutes, turning halfway through, until lightly browned on each side.
- In a blender, combine 1 of the bananas, the rice milk, almond butter, maple syrup, vanilla, cinnamon, nutmeg, and ⅛ teaspoon salt. Puree until smooth. Transfer the mixture to a large bowl.
- Warm the olive oil in a large nonstick skillet over medium-high heat. Dip the toasted bread slices into the mixture, turning so both sides absorb the liquid. Immediately place in the skillet and cook until golden brown on both sides, about 5 minutes total. Repeat with the remaining slices, adding more oil to the skillet as needed.
- For each serving, transfer 2 slices of French toast to a plate and drizzle the blueberry coulis over and around it. Garnish with the blueberries, strawberries, bananas slices, and toasted almonds. Serve immediately while they're still nice and crisp (or make in batches to order).

Potato Pancakes

PREPARATION TIME: 10 minutes
COOKING TIME: 30 minutes
YIELD: About 8 to 12 pancakes

3 tablespoons rice milk

¼ ripe banana, chopped

1 pound Yukon gold potatoes, peeled and coarsely grated

¼ cup grated red onion

3 tablespoons whole-wheat pastry flour

1 teaspoon baking powder

Coarse sea salt

Freshly ground black pepper

¼ teaspoon paprika

3 tablespoons extra-virgin olive oil, plus more as needed

Applesauce, for serving

- In a blender, puree the rice milk and banana. Set aside.
- Preheat the oven to 200°F.
- Drain the potatoes and onions by wrapping them in a clean dishtowel and wringing out the excess liquid. In a large bowl, combine the potatoes, onions, flour, baking powder, 1 teaspoon salt, ¼ teaspoon black pepper, the paprika, and the banana–rice milk mixture. Warm the olive oil in a large nonstick skillet over medium-high heat. Working in batches of 4, spoon 2 tablespoons of the potato mixture into the oil and flatten to about a 2 ½-inch diameter with a slotted spatula. Cook until golden brown on both sides, about 7 minutes total. Transfer the pancakes to paper towels to drain. Repeat with the remaining potato mixture, adding more oil to the skillet as necessary.
- Place the pancakes on a baking sheet and keep them warm in the oven until you're ready to serve. Serve with applesauce.

Sunflower Sprouts and Mixed Baby Greens Salad with Yogurt Dressing

PREPARATION TIME: 5 minutes

Sunflower sprouts are rich in chlorophyll, vitamins A, B$_1$, B$_2$, C, niacin, and the minerals calcium, magnesium, and potassium, so this simple salad adds green color and concentrated nutrients to the buffet.

2½ cups sunflower sprouts
1 pound mixed baby greens
2 tablespoons fresh lemon juice
1 small garlic clove, minced
Coarse sea salt and freshly ground white pepper
1 teaspoon Dijon mustard
¾ cup plain soy yogurt

- In a large salad bowl, combine the sunflower sprouts with the mixed baby greens and toss well.
- In a medium bowl, combine the lemon juice, garlic, salt to taste, pepper to taste, and the mustard. Whisk in the yogurt and transfer to a small serving bowl. Serve salad with dressing on the side.

Stone Fruit Salad

■ ■ ■

PREPARATION TIME: 15 minutes
INACTIVE PREPARATION TIME: 1 hour

Juicy fruit.

½ pound fresh cherries, pitted and halved
3 nectarines, pitted and cut into eighths
3 peaches, pitted and cut into eighths
6 plums, pitted and cut into fourths
1 teaspoon fresh lemon juice

■ In a large bowl, combine all the ingredients. Toss lightly, cover, and refrigerate for 1 hour.

Straight-Edge Tangerine Mimosa

■ ■ ■

PREPARATION TIME: 5 minutes

Fresh tangerine juice
Sparkling water
Tangerine slices, for garnish

■ Fill champagne flutes or glasses halfway with tangerine juice. Top with sparkling water. Garnish each serving with a tangerine slice and serve immediately.

Food for Thought

Reminisce about the days of your youth and give today's kids a break.

▌TIPS FOR PREPARING THIS MENU▐

The day before

- Roast the yellow peppers, cover with olive oil, and refrigerate.
- Make the tempeh sausage batter and store, covered, in the refrigerator.
- Make the coulis and store, covered, in the refrigerator. Reheat before serving and thin out with water if necessary.
- Make the yogurt dressing.

A few hours before

- Toast the bread for the French toast.
- Wash and spin dry the salad greens, cover with a damp towel and refrigerate.
- Make the stone fruit salad.
- Squeeze the tangerine juice.

At the meal

- Lay out a nice buffet for friends to enjoy. You can make the French toast on demand so each serving will be hot and fresh.

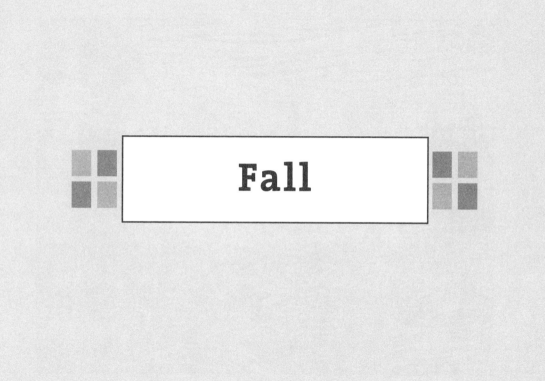

Fall

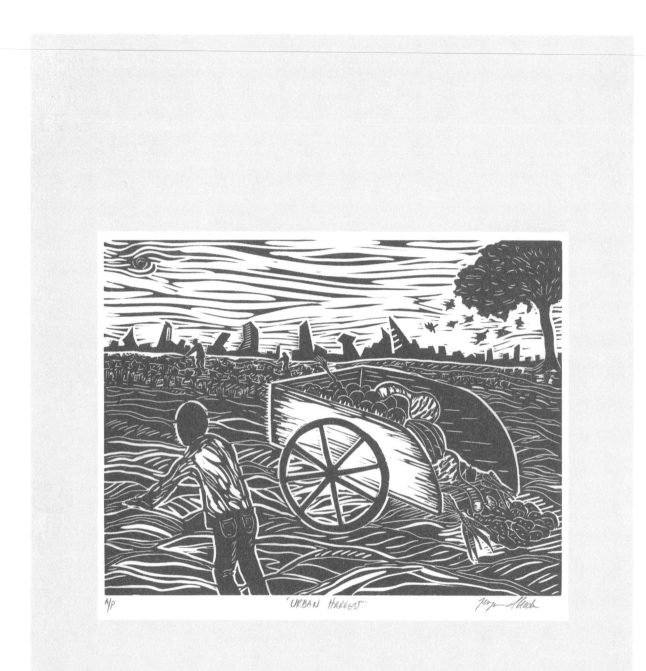

A/P   "URBAN HARVEST"

AFTER-DINNER DESSERT BUFFET

▪▪▪

Blood Orange Sorbet

▪

Black and Blue Berry Crisp

▪

Chocolate–Pecan Pudding Pie with Nut Crust

▪▪▪

Soundtrack
(provided by DJ Reborn)

D'Angelo, *Brown Sugar*
Dionne Farris, *Wild Seed Wild Flower*
Kim Hill, *Suga Hill*
Ohio Players, *Honey*
Lewis Taylor, *Lewis Taylor*

▪▪▪

Ma'Dear, my maternal grandmother, worked in her backyard garden with pure passion. The garden wasn't very large—probably the size of a built-in swimming pool—but it produced enough food for her to feed herself, Granddaddy, and her four grandchildren that she cared for during the summers. Ma'Dear made sure that she had enough food from April to November and plenty to preserve and freeze for the winter. In the kitchen, she kept a cupboard about seven feet tall and a foot deep, each shelf crowded with glass jars full of preserves: pickled pears, peaches, green tomatoes, carrots, and green beans; apples and figs, sauerkraut, and blackberry jam; and her not-to-be-forgotten chow chow—cabbage, peppers, green tomatoes, and onions finely chopped, cooked for five hours and served with leafy greens such as collards, mustards, or turnips.

And yes, Ma'Dear could throw down with the best of them. Upon entering her house, you knew she was cooking, even if you didn't smell it, because you'd hear singing:

Glory, glory, hallelujah.
When I lay my burden down.
No more Monday.
No more Tuesday.
When I lay my burden down.

Whenever she created her mouthwatering desserts, Ma'Dear would hum gospel songs and spirituals while rhythmically tapping her feet, sending music vibrating throughout the rooms of her house. When she rolled out the dough for her fried pies and sang those lines, it was as if her love and spirituality were two more ingredients she added, along with the flour, salt, lard, and water.

I lovingly created this menu with my sweet grandmothers, Margie Bryant (Ma'Dear) and Rosa Lee Terry (Granny), in mind.

These desserts can be enjoyed together as a buffet or individually with other menus in this book.

Blood Orange Sorbet

PREPARATION TIME: 20 minutes
INACTIVE PREPARATION TIME: Overnight plus 2 hours
YIELD: 1 quart

This sorbet is a great palate cleanser, and the Grand Marnier gives it spirit.

10 large blood oranges
½ cup organic raw cane sugar
¼ cup Grand Marnier

- With a serrated knife, peel the blood oranges, removing all the white pith. Segment the blood oranges, discarding the membrane and any seeds. Spread evenly on a tray that fits into the freezer. Partially freeze and then transfer to a container, cover, and freeze overnight.

- Make a simple syrup by combining ½ cup water with the sugar in a small saucepan over low heat. Stir well until hot to the touch and the sugar is completely dissolved. Remove from the heat.

- Add the Grand Marnier to the simple syrup and stir well. Cool completely.

- Break up the orange segments and, in a food processor, combine the frozen blood oranges with the simple syrup. Puree until smooth. Strain through a large-mesh strainer, transfer to a 1-quart container, cover, and freeze until firm, about 2 hours.

Black and Blue Berry Crisp

PREPARATION TIME: 15 minutes
COOKING TIME: 40 minutes
SERVES: 8

This is a great way to get the most out of seasonal fresh berries. I recommend vanilla ice cream to set this dessert off.

FRUIT

3 cups fresh blackberries
3 cups fresh blueberries
1 cup apple juice
2 tablespoons pure maple syrup
2 tablespoons organic raw cane sugar
½ teaspoon lemon zest
1 teaspoon fresh lemon juice

½ teaspoon ground ginger

Fine sea salt

2 tablespoons arrowroot

TOPPING

½ cup melted coconut oil

⅓ cup pure maple syrup

½ cup chopped walnuts

½ cup whole-wheat pastry flour

2 cups rolled oats

1 teaspoon ground cinnamon

½ teaspoon freshly grated nutmeg

Fine sea salt

FOR THE FRUIT

- Preheat the oven to 375°F.
- Place the blackberries and blueberries in a large bowl. In a separate bowl combine the apple juice, maple syrup, sugar, lemon zest, lemon juice, ginger, and a pinch of salt. Whisk in the arrowroot and pour over the berry mixture.

FOR THE TOPPING

- In a small bowl, combine the coconut oil and maple syrup and whisk well. In a separate bowl, combine the walnuts, flour, oats, cinnamon, nutmeg, and ¼ teaspoon salt. Mix well and add the coconut oil-maple syrup mixture. Toss well until combined.
- Transfer the berry filling to a 9x13-inch baking dish and evenly sprinkle the topping over the berries. Bake for 10 minutes, then lower the oven temperature to 350°F and bake another 20 to 25 minutes, or until the topping is golden and the filling is bubbling.
- Serve warm with vanilla ice cream.

Chocolate–Pecan Pudding Pie with Nut Crust

■ ■ ■

PREPARATION TIME: 15 minutes
INACTIVE PREPARATION TIME: 2 hours
COOKING TIME: 40 minutes

Coming home from Memphis a few years ago, I stumbled on an immediately mouthwatering recipe for Chocolate Pecan Pie (in of all places the airport!). The recipe had all the usual unhealthy trappings of Southern food: lots of "bad" fat and highly processed sugars. But by the time I got home, I had figured out which health-supportive ingredients could be substituted for the less healthy ones. I decided to use maple syrup, for instance, instead of light corn syrup. In the end, the only resemblance my pie had with the original one was the chocolate and pecans.

NUT CRUST

1 cup almonds

1 cup pecans

½ cup whole-wheat pastry flour

Fine sea salt

½ cup dried unsweetened coconut

8 large dates, pitted and chopped

¼ cup coconut oil

FILLING

¾ cup soymilk

¼ cup arrowroot

½ ripe banana

¾ cup chocolate chips

½ cup pure maple syrup

1 teaspoon pure vanilla extract

½ cup melted coconut oil

1¼ cups pecans, chopped
½ cup dried unsweetened coconut
Mint leaves, for garnish

FOR THE CRUST

- Preheat the oven to 325°F.
- Combine the almonds, pecans, flour, and ⅛ teaspoon salt in a food processor fitted with the metal blade and grind to a fine meal. Transfer to a large bowl and add the coconut. Add the dates and coconut oil to the food processor and process until the dates form into a gooey mass, about 1 minute. Add the dry ingredients back into the food processor and process until everything is mixed well and starts to form into a ball.
- Transfer the dough to a 9-inch pie tin. With clean hands, knead the dough for a minute or so to ensure that the oil is evenly distributed. Press the dough into the pan, making sure that the bottom, sides, and rim are covered (the sides should be slightly thicker than the bottom). With a fork, prick several holes into the bottom of the crust. Set aside.

FOR THE FILLING

- In a blender, combine the soymilk and arrowroot and puree for 30 seconds. Add the banana and puree for another 15 seconds. Set aside.
- In the top of a double boiler over simmering water, melt the chocolate chips. In a large bowl, immediately combine the melted chocolate chips with the soymilk mixture, maple syrup, vanilla, coconut oil, pecans, and coconut. Mix well. Scrape the filling into the crust with a rubber spatula and spread evenly.
- Place the pie on a cookie sheet. Cover the crust with aluminum foil and bake for about 20 minutes, until filling is firm.
- Remove from the oven, cool for 30 minutes, then refrigerate for at least 2 hours before serving.
- Garnish each slice with a few mint leaves.

Food for Thought

Remember all the ways that sweetness enters your life!

▪ TIPS FOR PREPARING THIS MENU ▪

- Freeze the blood oranges for the sorbet overnight.
- Pull the sorbet out of the freezer 10 to 15 minutes before serving to soften it.
- Time the cooking of the crisp so that it's done right before serving and folks can eat it hot.
- Buy vanilla ice cream to go with your crisp.
- Make the pie the day before and refrigerate overnight.

¡Grub Latinoamericano!

■ ■ ■

Baby Bella Mushroom Quesadillas

■

Smoky South American Seitan Stew

■

Coconut-Infused Quinoa

■

Green Cabbage Salad with Lime-Cilantro Vinaigrette

■ ■ ■

Soundtrack
(provided by Annemarie Colbin)

Antonio Carlos Jobim, *The Girl from Ipanema: The Antonio Carlos Jobim Songbook*
Astor Piazzolla, *The Best of Astor Piazzolla*
Astor Piazzolla, *Tango: Zero Hour*
Maria Dolores Pradera, *Ellas Cantan Asi*
Trio Los Panchos, *Love Songs of the Tropics*

■ ■ ■

I dedicate this menu to my friend Annemarie Colbin, founder of the Natural Gourmet Cookery School. Founded in 1977, it is the oldest natural foods cooking school in the United States. Annemarie was born in Holland but grew up in Argentina, where she became a vegetarian and started her journey studying the effects of food on health and inspiring people to cook delicious, health-supportive food.

Baby Bella Mushroom Quesadillas

■■■

PREPARATION TIME: 10 minutes
COOKING TIME: 20 minutes

1 tablespoon extra-virgin olive oil, plus more for cooking the tortillas
½ cup diced onions
Coarse sea salt
3 cups (about 10 ounces whole) cleaned, stemmed, and sliced Baby
    Bella mushrooms (or portobello mushrooms)
2 limes
Four 8-inch whole wheat tortillas
½ cup grated pepper jack cheese
1 jalapeño chile, seeded and finely chopped
Sour cream, for garnish
Cilantro sprigs, for garnish
Some good hot sauce, for serving

- Preheat the oven to 200°F.
- Warm 1 tablespoon of the olive oil in a large nonstick skillet over medium heat. Add the onions and ½ teaspoon salt. Sauté for 3 minutes, or until softened, stirring often. Add the mushrooms and sauté for an additional 4 minutes, or until they soften, stirring often. Squeeze 1 tablespoon of lime juice over the mixture and cook for 1 more minute. Transfer the mixture to a small bowl.
- Reduce the heat under the skillet just used to medium-low and warm 1 teaspoon of the olive oil. Add 1 tortilla and move it around to make sure it's covered with oil. Sprinkle 2 tablespoons of cheese on the bottom half of the tortilla. Add ¼ cup of the onion-mushroom mixture on top of that, followed by a quarter of the jalapeño, then squeeze a little lime juice over everything. Cook for 2 minutes, then fold the tortilla over and press down with a spatula for 15 seconds. Flip over and cook another 30 seconds. The quesadilla should be lightly browned on both sides.

- Place the quesadilla on a baking sheet and place in the oven to keep warm.
- Repeat to make 4 quesadillas, placing them in the oven as they are finished.
- Before serving, cut each quesadilla in half and serve on a large plate garnished with sour cream and cilantro. I like to open each one up and give it a dash of hot sauce.

Smoky South American Seitan Stew

PREPARATION TIME: 20 minutes
COOKING TIME: 1 hour and 10 minutes

I think chipotles were just made for this stew, which was inspired by one of chef Rick Bayless's seafood stews. The smoky-sweet flavor of the chipotles might catch some of your guests off guard at first, but they'll soon take pleasure in the combination of flavors.

5 tablespoons extra-virgin olive oil
1 cup thinly sliced red onions
1 chipotle chile, canned in adobo sauce, finely chopped
10 garlic cloves, roughly chopped
One 28-ounce can whole tomatoes, drained
2 bay leaves
4 cups vegetable stock
Coarse sea salt
3 medium red potatoes (about 1 pound),
    scrubbed and cut into ½-inch pieces
8 ounces seitan, cut into ¼-inch slices
2 large ripe plantains, cut diagonally into ½-inch slices
½ cup chopped fresh cilantro

- Combine 2 tablespoons of the olive oil with the onions and chipotles in a medium saucepan over high heat and cook for 2 minutes, stirring frequently. Reduce the heat to low and cook uncovered for 10 minutes, stirring occasionally. Add the garlic and cook for 5 more minutes.

- Transfer the mixture to a blender, add the tomatoes, and puree until smooth. Pour the mixture back in the saucepan, add the bay leaves, and stir constantly over medium heat until cooked down to a thick consistency, about 10 minutes. Stir in the vegetable stock and 1 teaspoon salt, plus more to taste if needed.

- Add the potatoes and seitan, bring to a boil, cover the pot, reduce the heat to low, and simmer for 45 minutes, or until the potatoes have softened and the stew has thickened somewhat. Remove the bay leaves.

- Meanwhile, warm the remaining 3 tablespoons olive oil in a large frying pan over medium heat. Add the plantains (in batches if necessary) and fry until golden brown, 2 to 3 minutes on each side. Drain the plantains on paper towels.

- Add the plantains and cilantro to the stew and simmer for 5 more minutes.

Coconut-Infused Quinoa

PREPARATION TIME: 5 minutes
COOKING TIME: 25 minutes

This ancient South American cereal grain is higher in protein than any other grain. It tastes great cooked in coconut milk, and it's heavenly after soaking up some of the smoky stew.

1 cup coconut milk, fresh (see page 252) or canned
Coarse sea salt
1 cup quinoa
2 tablespoons dried unsweetened coconut

- Combine the coconut milk with 1 cup water and ½ teaspoon salt in a medium saucepan over high heat and bring to a boil. Add the quinoa and dried coconut, bring back to a boil, then reduce the heat, cover the pot, and simmer for 20 minutes. Remove from the heat and steam with lid on for 5 minutes, then lightly fluff with a fork.

Green Cabbage Salad with Lime-Cilantro Vinaigrette

■ ■ ■

PREPARATION TIME: 10 minutes

INACTIVE PREPARATION TIME: 30 minutes to overnight

This is a great raw salad for the winter months. It's perfect for balancing out this menu's heavy stew. And did you know that cabbage is higher in vitamin C than oranges?

DRESSING
2 tablespoons fresh lime juice

1 teaspoon Dijon mustard

1 tablespoon minced fresh cilantro

2 teaspoons pure maple syrup

Coarse sea salt

3 tablespoons extra-virgin olive oil

SALAD
5 cups thinly sliced green cabbage (about ¾ small head)

1 jalapeño chile, seeded and finely chopped

1 small radish, thinly sliced, for garnish

- In a blender, combine the lime juice, mustard, cilantro, maple syrup, and 1 teaspoon salt. Blend while slowly pouring in the oil.
- Place the cabbage in a large bowl and add the vinaigrette. With clean hands, massage the cabbage for 3 to 5 minutes, thoroughly coating it with the vinaigrette. Add the jalapeño, mix well (not with your hands), cover, and chill for at least 30 minutes, or overnight. Remove from the refrigerator 10 minutes before serving, and garnish with radish slices.

Food for Thought

Remember, with the use of best-quality ingredients, health-supportive cooking techniques, and your positive energy, a lot of food can be Grub.

TIPS FOR PREPARING THIS MENU

- If possible, make the stew the night before. It will be much more flavorful.
- Prep the ingredients for the quesadillas a few hours before.
- Make the salad, cover, and refrigerate it overnight.

More Than One Side (Dish) to Thanksgiving

■ ■ ■

Mac 4 Cheese (with Leeks)

■

Apple-Cranberry Sauce

■

Roasted Yam Puree with Coconut Milk

■

Brussels Sprouts with White Wine and Thyme

■

Frankie and Anna's Walnut-Cheddar Casserole

■

Rosemary-Butter Biscuits

■ ■ ■

Soundtrack

(provided by Evon Peter)

Blackfire, *One Nation Under*
Buffy Sainte-Marie, *Native North American Child: An Odyssey*
Pamyua, *Menglini*
Ras K'dee, *Street Prison*
Ras K'dee, *Transcendental State of Music*

■ ■ ■

When I was growing up, Thanksgiving was *the* family gathering of the year. We would all meet at my grandparents' house for the whole day and feast. The meals were always potluck—my grandparents would cook turkey, ham, and roast beef, and everyone else would bring side dishes to create an oversized buffet. This was not built as a complete menu. Since so many celebrate Thanksgiving with extended family members, I offer you several casual side dishes to add some variety to this year's menu. These recipes can be doubled for bigger gatherings.

Mac 4 Cheese (with Leeks)

PREPARATION TIME: 20 minutes
COOKING TIME: About 1 hour

This is a lovely reinvention of the macaroni and cheese that my mom made when I was growing up. With leeks, too.

Coarse salt
2 cups uncooked whole-wheat elbow macaroni
5 tablespoons extra-virgin olive oil
2 thinly sliced large leeks, white and light green parts only (see Box)
3 tablespoons whole-wheat flour
3 cups whole milk
1 tablespoon white balsamic vinegar
½ teaspoon paprika
Pinch of cayenne
1 cup grated cheddar cheese
1 cup grated pepper jack cheese
½ cup grated fresh mozzarella
½ cup freshly grated Parmesan cheese
Freshly ground black pepper
2 tablespoons chopped fresh rosemary

- Preheat the oven to 375°F and lightly grease a shallow 2-quart baking dish.
- Bring a large pot of water to a boil for the pasta. Add 2 teaspoons salt. When the

water returns to a boil, stir in the pasta and cook until al dente, about 6 minutes. Drain the pasta and set aside.

- Meanwhile, in a medium sauté pan over medium heat, warm 2 tablespoons of the olive oil. Add the leeks and ½ teaspoon salt. Sauté for 5 to 7 minutes, until the leeks are lightly browned. Remove from the heat and set aside.

- Warm the remaining 3 tablespoons olive oil in a medium saucepan over medium-low heat and whisk in the flour. Cook for 3 to 4 minutes, whisking every 30 seconds, until the flour is a darker shade of brown.

- Raise the heat to medium, add the milk, and bring to a simmer, whisking constantly. Simmer for 10 minutes, whisking constantly, until thickened.

- Reduce the heat to low, add the vinegar, paprika, cayenne, ½ teaspoon salt, ½ cup of the cheddar, ½ cup of the pepper jack, the mozzarella, and Parmesan to the white sauce and stir until smooth. Season with black pepper to taste.

- Add the leeks and elbows to the white sauce, gently stir well, and pour into the baking dish.

- Sprinkle the remaining ½ cup cheddar and ½ cup pepper jack over the top and garnish with the chopped rosemary.

- Bake for 35 to 40 minutes, until lightly browned and crisp on top. Serve hot.

CLEANING LEEKS

First cut off the greens, leaving only the light green and white bottom, then cut off the roots. Slice the leek in half lengthwise, then thinly slice it horizontally. Fill a large bowl with cold water. Add the leek slices, and swish around well, vigorously, rubbing any dirt and sand off the pieces. Lift from the water and set in a colander. Rinse the bowl of any residue and repeat if necessary.

Apple-Cranberry Sauce

PREPARATION TIME: 10 minutes
COOKING TIME: 10 minutes

After trying this cranberry sauce you'll never eat canned cranberry sauce again. This version, using fresh cranberries, apples, and tangerine juice, is so naturally sweet and yummy you could even eat it as dessert.

1 cup fresh cranberries
1 cup peeled and diced sweet-tart apples such as Braeburn, Early Crisp,
*   or Gala*
½ cup fresh tangerine juice (or fresh orange juice)
2 tablespoons organic raw cane sugar
Pinch of fine sea salt
Pinch of ground ginger
Pinch of ground cinnamon

- Combine all the ingredients in a medium saucepan over medium heat and bring to a boil. Reduce the heat and simmer for 10 minutes, stirring every 2 minutes, until soft with some chunks remaining. Remove from the heat, cool to room temperature, and refrigerate. Serve cool.

Roasted Yam Puree with Coconut Milk

■■■

PREPARATION TIME: 15 minutes
COOKING TIME: 40 minutes

This dish is creamy orange bliss. Often confused with sweet potatoes, yams contain more natural sugar and have a higher moisture content. When buying yams, select smaller ones (they're sweeter) and ones that are unwrinkled with few blemishes. If you can't find yams, you can substitute sweet potatoes.

4 pounds yams, peeled and cut into 1-inch chunks
4 tablespoons pure maple syrup
6 tablespoons extra-virgin olive oil
Coarse sea salt
½ cup coconut milk, fresh (see page 252), or canned, warmed,
  plus more if needed

- Preheat the oven to 375°F. Lightly oil a baking dish or roasting pan.
- In a large bowl, combine the yams, maple syrup, olive oil, and ½ teaspoon sea salt. Toss well.
- Transfer the yams to the prepared pan and roast for 40 minutes, stirring every 10 minutes, until slightly crisp on the edges.
- Remove from the oven. In a food processor, combine the yams with the warmed coconut milk. Puree, adding more coconut milk for your desired consistency, and transfer to a serving dish.

Brussels Sprouts with
White Wine and Thyme

■ ■ ■

PREPARATION TIME: 15 minutes
COOKING TIME: 10 minutes

Unfortunately, a lot of people have bad childhood memories of being forced to eat over-cooked, bitter Brussels sprouts. So I have to be very careful when describing this dish: "So, you like white wine, right?" "How do you feel about thyme?" "What if you combined them with some fresh baby cabbages?" Try to repress any personal Brussels sprouts trauma, and give these baby cabbages a try.

2 tablespoons extra-virgin olive oil

1 pound Brussels sprouts, stems trimmed and cut in half lengthwise

3 garlic cloves, minced

7 to 8 fresh thyme sprigs

½ cup vegetable stock

½ cup white wine

Coarse sea salt

Freshly ground white pepper

■   Coat a large sauté pan with the olive oil. Add the Brussels sprouts, arranging them cut side down in one snug layer. Turn the heat to high and sauté until the cut side of the Brussels sprouts are lightly browned, 2 to 3 minutes. Add the garlic and thyme. Sauté for about 2 minutes, or until the garlic is fragrant, stirring to evenly distribute the garlic and thyme. Add the vegetable stock, wine, and 1 teaspoon salt. Bring to a boil and stir well. Immediately lower the heat to low, cover, and braise until the Brussels sprouts are tender, about 7 minutes. Remove from the heat and remove the thyme stems.

■   Season with additional salt and white pepper to taste and serve hot.

Frankie and Anna's
Walnut-Cheddar Casserole

PREPARATION TIME: 15 minutes
COOKING TIME: 30 minutes

This dish, adapted from Frances Moore Lappé's *Diet for a Small Planet,* complements these sides, and it's easy to make.

CASSEROLE

2 tablespoons olive oil

2 cups chopped onions

1 cup chopped black walnuts (black walnuts are more flavorful, but if
    you can't find them, regular walnuts will do)

2 tablespoons fresh lemon juice

2 large eggs, beaten

Coarse sea salt

2 tablespoons nutritional yeast

1 teaspoon caraway seeds

1 ¼ cups cooked brown rice (from ½ cup uncooked)
    (see page 146)

SAUCE

2 tablespoons unsalted butter

2 tablespoons whole wheat pastry flour

½ cup vegetable stock

1 cup milk

½ cup shredded cheddar cheese

Coarse sea salt

Freshly ground black pepper

FOR THE CASSEROLE

- Preheat the oven to 350°F. Oil an 8½ x 4½ x 2¾-inch loaf pan.
- Heat the oil in a large sauté pan over medium heat. Add the onions and sauté until translucent, about 8 to 10 minutes. Mix in the remaining casserole ingredients and transfer to the prepared pan. Bake for 30 minutes, or until firm and slightly browned.

FOR THE SAUCE

- While the loaf is baking make the sauce. Melt the butter in a medium saucepan over medium heat. Stir in the flour and cook, stirring, for 1½ minutes, or until fragrant.
- Add the vegetable stock and milk and stir well. Add the cheese and simmer until it starts to thicken, about 3 to 5 minutes. Add ½ teaspoon salt and black pepper to taste. Remove from the heat and serve a dollop with each slice.

Rosemary-Butter Biscuits

PREPARATION TIME: 15 minutes
COOKING TIME: 15 minutes

¾ cup whole-wheat pastry flour

1¼ cups unbleached all-purpose flour

1 tablespoon organic raw cane sugar

4 teaspoons baking powder

Fine sea salt

2 tablespoons fresh minced rosemary

6 tablespoons cold unsalted butter, cut into bits, plus more for serving

¾ cup organic whole milk

- Preheat the oven to 400°F.
- Sift the flours, sugar, baking powder, and ½ teaspoon salt into a large bowl. Stir in the rosemary. With a pastry cutter or fork, cut the butter into the dry ingredients until the mixture looks like coarse cornmeal.
- Add the milk all at once and mix with a large spoon just until the dough forms into a ball. With lightly floured hands, knead the dough on a lightly floured surface just a couple of times, until it all comes together.
- Roll out the dough about ½ inch thick, and then cut with a 2-inch biscuit cutter or drinking glass. Place the biscuits on an ungreased baking sheet a few inches apart from each other. Bake until the biscuits are golden brown on top, about 15 minutes.
- Remove from oven, cut a widthwise slit halfway into each biscuit and add a thin sliver of butter. Serve hot.

Food for Thought

During Thanksgiving, be mindful of the Native people of North America and all their historical and contemporary struggles.

TIPS FOR PREPARING THIS MENU

- Roast the yams and make the Mac 4 Cheese at the same time.
- The Apple-Cranberry Sauce can be made the day before and kept refrigerated.

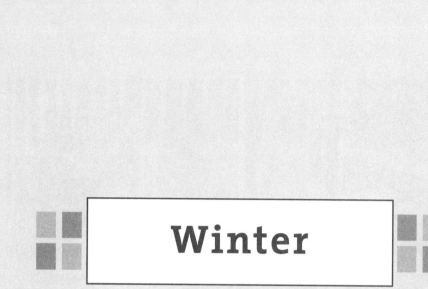

Winter

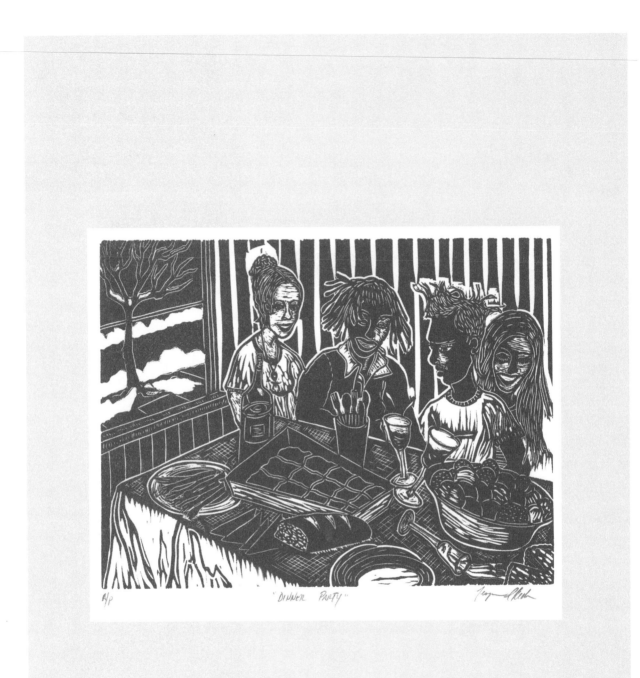

A/P   "DINNER PARTY"

New Year's Eve Good Luck Hors D'oeuvres

■ ■ ■

Winter Crudités with Hummus

■

Mini-Black-Eyed Pea and Goober Croquettes with
Yogurt-Dill Dip

■

Quinoa–Stuffed Cabbage Packages

■

Cinnamon-Dusted Sweet Potato Fries

■

Money Green Champagne

Note about serving size: This menu is designed for a party of 8 to 10 people.

■ ■ ■

Soundtrack

Césaria Évora, *Club Sodade*
Cottonbelly, *NYC Sessions 1993–2004: X Amounts Of Niceness*
DJ Kicks—Daddy G (Compilation)
M.I.A., *Arular*
Phat Global #1 (Compilation)

■ ■ ■

One custom dear to my paternal grandfather, Paw Paw, was eating a "New Year's Good Luck Meal," a ritual among many Southerners that dates back to the antebellum period. Although it differs in various parts of the South, it always includes two key staples: black-eyed peas, and either cabbage or turnip greens. In Southern lore, the peas represent copper and turnips and cabbage represent the almighty dollar. Other side dishes and bread might be included to round off the meal, and many older folks will include some part of the pig (ham, hog's jowls, or the whole hog's head).

Paw Paw's version consisted of the following: a gigantic pot of black-eyed peas cooked for several hours and seasoned with hearty chunks of ham and lard; green cabbage leaves sautéed until they were limp and beige; baked chunks of sweet potatoes seasoned with brown sugar and cinnamon; black-iron-skillet cornbread; and an oven-baked hogshead.

My father has carried on this tradition for as long as I can remember. He and my mother used to buy a piece of hog's head to eat on New Year's Day, but they embraced a healthier diet after I was born and cut out a lot of pork products. In that spirit, I used the same staples and reinvented this meal to suit more modern tastes and health concerns.

Anna and I wish you and your loved ones a prosperous New Year.

Winter Crudités with Hummus

■ ■ ■

PREPARATION TIME: 20 minutes

HUMMUS
4 cups cooked chickpeas (from 1⅓ cups dried chickpeas), drained,
with cooking liquid reserved (or two 16-ounce cans of
cooked chickpeas)
¼ cup tahini
¼ cup fresh lemon juice, or to taste
2 garlic cloves, minced
½ teaspoon ground cumin
Coarse sea salt
½ cup extra-virgin olive oil, plus more for drizzling

Freshly ground black pepper

Paprika, for sprinkling

CRUDITÉS

8 slices pita bread

Extra-virgin olive oil, for drizzling

8 medium carrots, peeled and cut into 4-inch sticks

2 medium daikon radishes, peeled and cut into 4-inch sticks

2 bunches radishes (about 20), tops and ends trimmed and quartered

FOR THE HUMMUS

- In a food processor or blender, combine the chickpeas, tahini, lemon juice, garlic, cumin, and ¾ teaspoon salt. Puree until smooth, adding the olive oil through the machine's feed tube. Add some chickpea cooking liquid (or water if using canned chickpeas) if necessary to achieve a smooth consistency. Add additional salt and black pepper to taste.
- Transfer to a serving bowl. Drizzle with olive oil and sprinkle with paprika.

FOR THE CRUDITÉS

- Preheat the oven to 350°F.
- Stack the pita bread into two stacks of four. With a large serrated knife, cut each stack like pizza into eight wedges. Lay them in a single layer on large baking sheets. Bake until lightly toasted, turning once, about 10 minutes total. Drizzle with olive oil.
- Place the bowl of hummus on the center of a plate and artfully place the vegetables and pita bread around it. Serve at room temperature.

Mini-Black-Eyed Pea and Goober Croquettes with Yogurt-Dill Dip

■■■

PREPARATION TIME: 45 minutes
INACTIVE PREPARATION TIME: Overnight
COOKING TIME: 1 hour and 10 minutes
YIELD: About 32 croquettes

Full of black-eyed peas and goobers (a Southern word for peanuts), these tasty croquettes should please your palate and bring lots of good luck.

DIP
1½ cups plain yogurt
2 tablespoons chopped fresh dill
½ teaspoon coarse sea salt
1 teaspoon fresh lemon juice
Freshly ground black pepper

CROQUETTES
1¼ cups black-eyed peas, sorted, soaked overnight,
*   drained, and rinsed*
1 tablespoon plus ½ teaspoon extra-virgin olive oil, plus more if frying
Coarse sea salt
1 medium green bell pepper, seeded and finely chopped
1 medium red onion, finely chopped
1 teaspoon chili powder
½ teaspoon ground cumin
Pinch of cayenne pepper
¼ cup unsalted peanuts, chopped
2 garlic cloves, minced
2 teaspoons balsamic vinegar

2 tablespoons fresh lemon juice

1 tablespoon chickpea miso

About ½ cup whole-wheat breadcrumbs

FOR THE DIP

- Combine all the dip ingredients in a medium bowl and stir well. Set aside while you prepare the croquettes.

FOR THE CROQUETTES

- Combine the black-eyed peas with 5 cups of water and ½ teaspoon of the olive oil in a medium saucepan over medium heat and bring to a boil. Skim off any foam, reduce the heat to medium-low, and simmer, partially covered, for 15 minutes. Add 1 teaspoon salt and simmer for another 15 minutes, until softened but still firm. Reserve ½ cup of the cooking liquid and set aside. Drain, rinse with cold water, and set aside.
- Preheat the oven to 350°F. Line a baking sheet with parchment paper.
- Combine 1 tablespoon of the olive oil, the bell pepper, onion, chili powder, cumin, cayenne, 1 teaspoon salt, and the peanuts in a large sauté pan over medium heat. Sauté for 8 minutes, or until the vegetables have softened. Add the garlic and cook for an additional 2 minutes.
- Stir the black-eyed peas into the mixture and cook for 3 additional minutes. Add the vinegar and lemon juice and cook for an additional minute.
- In a food processor, combine the mixture with the lemon juice and miso, and pulse just until it holds its shape, scraping down the sides a few times. Do not process until smooth—you should still have visible black-eyed pea pieces. Scrape the mixture into a large bowl and add breadcrumbs by the tablespoon until you've made a batter that is barely stiff enough to handle. Taste and add additional salt if necessary.
- Remove from the heat and cool slightly.
- Form the mixture into walnut-sized balls.
- Arrange the croquettes on the prepared baking sheet ½ inch apart. Slightly flatten each ball with a spatula and bake for about 20 minutes, carefully turning once, until golden brown on both sides.

- If you're not serving right away, keep the croquettes warm in the oven, lowering the oven temperature to 200°F.
- Place the yogurt-dill dip in a serving bowl on the center of a large serving plate. Artfully place the croquettes around it. The croquettes are fragile, so handle with care.

Quinoa–Stuffed Cabbage Packages

PREPARATION TIME: 10 minutes
COOKING TIME: 50 minutes
YIELD: 12 packages

Each cabbage leaf represents $1,000 that you will see in the New Year, so eat up.

1 cup quinoa
Coarse sea salt
1 large green cabbage head
12 chives
¼ cup extra-virgin olive oil
2 tablespoons fresh lime juice
4 tablespoons fresh orange juice
4 garlic cloves, minced and sautéed in olive oil
*   for 1 to 2 minutes until golden*
¼ cup currants
¼ cup toasted walnuts, chopped
3 tablespoons minced fresh parsley
Freshly ground white pepper

- If it is not prerinsed, rinse the quinoa in a fine-mesh strainer under running water and drain. Combine the quinoa, ½ teaspoon salt, and 2 cups of water in a large

- saucepan over high heat and bring to a boil. Reduce the heat to low, cover, and simmer for 20 minutes, until all of the water is absorbed. Let the quinoa steam with the top on for 15 minutes, then remove the top and cool.

- Meanwhile, bring a large deep pot of water to a boil and add 2 tablespoons salt. Prepare a large bowl full of ice water.

- Cut the core from the cabbage with a small paring knife. Drop the whole cabbage into the water and boil for 5 to 10 minutes, remove the cabbage head, and remove the softened outer leaves. Shock the leaves in the ice water to set the color and stop the cooking. Return the cabbage head to the boiling water to soften the next few layers of leaves, remove them, shock them, and continue with the rest of the cabbage. Drain and pat the cabbage leaves dry with paper towels. Set aside on paper towels.

- Bring the water back to a boil and add half of the chives. Blanch for 10 seconds, then remove them with tongs to the ice water. Drain and set aside on paper towels. Repeat with the remaining chives.

- In a large bowl combine the olive oil, lime juice, orange juice, garlic, currants, walnuts, and parsley. Mix well. Add the cooled quinoa and toss well with clean hands. Add ½ teaspoon salt, plus more to taste if needed. Add white pepper to taste.

- With a sharp knife, cut the thick part of the stem from each cabbage leaf. Place a heaping 3 tablespoons of the quinoa in the center of each cabbage leaf. Fold the sides toward the center and fold up each end of the leaf into a compact package. Wrap a chive around the narrower side of each package and tie it up into a knot.

- Serve on a large platter with the seam side facing down.

Cinnamon-Dusted Sweet Potato Fries

PREPARATION TIME: 10 minutes

INACTIVE PREPARATION TIME: At least 1 hour, or overnight

COOKING TIME: 30 minutes

We generally avoid deep-frying foods, but hey, it's New Year's Eve. And these fries are bangin'. Indulge a little. Organic coconut oil, which can be found in health food stores, is excellent for this dish.

4 large sweet potatoes (about 4 pounds), peeled

Coarse sea salt

Organic, unrefined coconut cooking oil, for frying

3 tablespoons ground cinnamon

- Cut the sweet potatoes into slices about ½ inch thick, then cut them lengthwise into the shape of slim fries.
- In a large bowl, combine the sweet potatoes with 1 teaspoon salt and enough cold water to cover by a few inches. Cover and refrigerate for at least 1 hour, or overnight.
- Thoroughly drain the sweet potatoes in a colander. Pat them well with paper towels until completely dry.
- Heat the coconut oil in a large saucepan or deep-fryer over medium-high heat until it reaches a temperature of 325°F, 6 to 8 minutes. Fry the potatoes, in batches, until lightly browned. Remove the fries from the oil with a slotted spoon or spider and place on a paper towel–lined plate. Increase the heat to high until it reaches 375°F, then add the par-fried potatoes, in batches, back into the oil and fry until crisp, 2 to 4 minutes. Again, remove the fries from the oil with a slotted spoon or spider and place on a paper towel–lined plate. Dust with cinnamon and serve immediately.

Money Green Champagne

PREPARATION TIME: 5 minutes

For playas only. Get ya drink on.

Leaves from 8 fresh mint sprigs
2 tablespoons organic raw cane sugar
2 tablespoons fresh lime juice
1 bottle chilled champagne

- In a mortar or suribachi, pulverize the mint with the sugar and lime juice.
- In a large bowl combine the mint mixture with the champagne (add the champagne slowly) and stir well.
- Strain the champagne into a large pitcher and serve immediately in champagne flutes.

Note: Cuvée Jean Louis from Charles de Fère, a luscious, creamy Blanc de Blancs Brut, is great for this drink.

> ## NOT-SO-OBVIOUS KITCHEN GEAR #4:
> ## MORTAR AND PESTLE
>
> Mortar and pestles have been used in cooking throughout the world, from the ancient Mayans to Southern African tribes. I have a collection from around the world in my kitchen.

TIPS FOR PREPARING THIS MENU

- Make the hummus the day before and refrigerate.
- Make the quinoa the day before and refrigerate.
- Soak the sweet potatoes in cold water overnight.

NEW MILLENNIUM SOUL FOOD

▪ ▪ ▪

Ginger Cornbread Muffins

▪

Spicy Barbecued Tofu Triangles

▪

Rosemary-Chile Mashed Potatoes

▪

Citrus Collards with Raisins

▪ ▪ ▪

Soundtrack
(provided by Jessica B. Harris)

Ray Charles, *The Very Best of Ray Charles*
Olu Dara, *In the World: From Natchez to New York*
Corey Harris, *Greens from the Garden*
Mahalia Jackson, *The World's Greatest Gospel Singer*
The Neville Brothers, *Treacherous: A History of the Neville Brothers*

▪ ▪ ▪

My father recently reminded me about the hours spent in my grandparents' garden when I was a child. Both of my grandfathers grew up in rural Mississippi, and they lived and worked on land owned by their families. Like the majority of Southern African-Americans of their generation who moved to urban centers like Memphis, they brought with them memories and survival skills of country living. Both sets of my grandparents had backyard gardens, and they grew most of their food—vegetables, fruits, and legumes (with the help of all their grandkids, of course). The only foods that they bought at the grocery store were meats, dried spices, fats for cooking, and flours for baking.

Paw Paw, my paternal grandfather, converted his whole half-acre backyard into a garden with little pathways leading to each tidy section. If you didn't work in Paw Paw's garden, you didn't eat, so his children, in-laws, and grandchildren worked in the garden as much as possible because Paw Paw was a gifted chef. We would help plant, tend, harvest, shell, shuck, snap, and eat everything from acorn squash to zucchini. And because he had a lot of surplus, Paw Paw also gave away several pounds of food to neighbors and church members. I like to think that we had our own community-supported agriculture (CSA) back then.

For this meal, I take family-favorite dishes and substitute more healthful ingredients and animal-free alternatives for the fatty meats more common to soul food. For example, I use a generous dose of chipotle chiles to give the barbecue sauce a smoky flavor and rosemary to make the mashed potatoes more fragrant. I also take collard greens, a Southern favorite, and offer a sweet lighter variation. I am happy to report that this meal has made it past the test of two of the most discriminating soul food connoisseurs I know—my parents.

Ginger Cornbread Muffins

■ ■ ■

PREPARATION TIME: 15 minutes
COOKING TIME: 25 minutes

Fresh ginger juice gives these cornbread muffins a spicy, sweet taste, and helps clear up any mid-winter congestion. These muffins also make nice breakfast treats with a little honey butter spread over them.

¾ cup yellow cornmeal
¾ cup all-purpose flour
1 tablespoon organic raw cane sugar
1 tablespoon baking powder
½ teaspoon ground cinnamon
Fine sea salt
¼ large ripe banana

¼ cup fresh ginger juice (from about 1 packed cup
    freshly grated ginger root) (see page 152)
1 cup plain soymilk
2 tablespoons pure maple syrup
3 tablespoons organic corn oil

- Set a rack in the middle of the oven. Preheat the oven to 350°F. Grease a 6-cup large muffin tin with corn oil.
- In a large bowl, whisk together the cornmeal, flour, sugar, baking powder, cinnamon, and ¾ teaspoon salt.
- In a large bowl, using a fork mash the banana with the ginger juice. Add the soymilk and mix until well combined. Add the maple syrup and corn oil and whisk well.
- Using a rubber spatula, fold the wet mixture into the dry mixture. Don't overmix, or the muffins will be dense.
- Spoon the batter into the muffin cups three-quarters full. Bake for 25 minutes, or until the tops are golden.
- Place a wet towel beneath the muffin pan and lift the muffins out.

Spicy Barbecued Tofu Triangles

PREPARATION TIME: 10 minutes
COOKING TIME: 1 hour and 40 minutes

This tasty barbecue sauce was inspired by a recipe from one of my favorite cookbooks, *The Modern Vegetarian Kitchen* by Peter Berley.

2 pounds extra-firm tofu (two large tofu cakes), pressed (see page 267)
6 tablespoons extra-virgin olive oil, plus more as needed
¼ cup apple cider vinegar

2 tablespoons fresh lime juice

¾ cup tamari

¼ cup canned tomato sauce

1 large chipotle chile, canned in adobo sauce

6 tablespoons pure maple syrup

2 teaspoons ground cumin

Pinch of cayenne pepper

- Preheat the oven to 350°F.
- Place each tofu cake on its side and cut into thirds. Keeping the layers together, cut the tofu diagonally to make 6 long triangles, then cut the triangles down the middle to make 12 smaller triangles. Pat each triangle well with paper towels.
- Warm 3 tablespoons olive oil in a large nonstick skillet over medium heat. Fry the tofu triangles in one snug layer, until golden brown, 7 to 10 minutes on each side, (adding more oil if needed), in batches if necessary. Drain the tofu triangles on paper towels.
- In a blender, combine the vinegar, lime juice, tamari, tomato sauce, chile, 3 tablespoons olive oil, maple syrup, cumin, cayenne, and 2 tablespoons water. Puree for 30 seconds, until smooth.
- Place the tofu in a large baking dish and cover with the marinade. Tightly cover the dish with foil. Bake for 1 hour, turning once halfway through.
- Transfer the tofu and the remaining marinade to a serving bowl, and serve with extra sauce spooned on top.

Rosemary-Chile Mashed Potatoes

■ ■ ■

PREPARATION TIME: 15 minutes
COOKING TIME: 25 minutes

The rosemary-chile oil gives these mashed potatoes just as much depth as butter. The rosemary also makes this dish deliciously fragrant, while the chile gives it some kick. This is one of the easiest side dishes to prepare—after you make the rosemary-chile oil, all you need to do is boil the potatoes, add the remaining ingredients, and mash.

ROSEMARY-CHILE OIL
1 cup extra-virgin olive oil
3 fresh rosemary sprigs
1 habanero chile, seeded and chopped

MASHED POTATOES
2 pounds Yukon gold potatoes, scrubbed well
¾ cup unflavored rice milk
1 tablespoon minced fresh rosemary
Coarse sea salt
Freshly ground white pepper

FOR THE ROSEMARY-CHILE OIL
- Combine the olive oil, rosemary sprigs, and chile in a small saucepan over high heat. When the rosemary sprigs begin to bubble, reduce the heat to low and simmer for 15 minutes.
- Remove the oil from the heat, let sit for 30 minutes, then strain into a glass jar.

TO MAKE THE MASHED POTATOES

- Combine the potatoes with cold water to cover by a few inches in a large pot over high heat. Bring to a rolling boil and cook until the potatoes can be easily pierced with a fork, about 25 minutes.
- Remove from the heat, drain, and peel the potatoes while they are still hot, hot, hot! Return them to the pot.
- Meanwhile, in a small saucepan over medium heat, combine ¼ cup of the rosemary-chile oil with the rice milk and bring to a simmer. (I use the leftover oil for dipping bread in or for pasta.)
- Add the rosemary-chile oil–rice milk mixture to the potatoes and mash well, until the potatoes are light and fluffy, adding more oil if needed. Add the chopped rosemary, 1½ teaspoons salt plus more to taste, and white pepper to taste.

Citrus Collards with Raisins

PREPARATION TIME: 10 minutes
COOKING TIME: 15 minutes

Though I love savory collard greens, I created this sweet, modern variation to be paired with savory entrées.

Coarse sea salt
2 large bunches collard greens, cut into chiffonade
*   (see page 145)*
1 tablespoon extra-virgin olive oil
2 garlic cloves, minced
⅔ cup raisins
⅓ cup fresh orange juice

- Bring 3 quarts of water to a boil in a large pot over high heat and add 1 tablespoon salt. Add the collards and cook, uncovered, for 8 to 10 minutes, until softened.
- Prepare a large bowl of ice water to cool the collards.
- Remove the collards from the heat, drain, and plunge them into the ice water to stop the cooking and to set the color. Drain.
- Warm the olive oil in a medium sauté pan over medium heat. Add the garlic and sauté for 1 minute. Add the collards, raisins, and a ½ teaspoon salt. Sauté for 3 minutes, stirring frequently, until the raisins are plump. Do not overcook—the collards should be bright green.
- Add the orange juice and cook for an additional 15 seconds. Season with additional salt to taste if needed and serve immediately.

▋ TIPS FOR PREPARING THIS MENU ▋

- Since this is a rich meal, you can add some mixed greens with a basic vinaigrette to lighten it up and introduce a raw element.
- Prepare the rosemary-chile oil a few days in advance.
- Make the barbecue sauce and cut the tofu into triangles. Add the tofu to the marinade and store, covered, in the refrigerator overnight.
- Wash the collards and cut into chiffonade a day in advance. Store them in a plastic bag in the refrigerator.

Mardi Gras Grub (Phat Tuesday)

■ ■ ■

Cajun-Spiced Tempeh Po' Boys (undressed)

■

Fresh Herb–Baked French Fries with Creole Mustard

■

Carrot Coleslaw

■

Frozen Blackberry Slurricane

■ ■ ■

Soundtrack
(provided by Bruce Mack)

The Dirty Dozen Brass Band, *This Is The Dirty Dozen Brass Band Collection*
Mardi Gras Classics (Compilation)
The Meters, *The Very Best of the Meters*
Rebirth Brass Band, *Hot Venom*
Ultimate Mardis Gras (Compilation)

We invite you to keep the spirit of New Orleans alive in your heart and kitchen.

■ ■ ■

DOWN IN NEW ORLEANS

Saffron skies
Chase down the sun
another seething day is done
Heat seasoned skin
keeps it hotter than the parish church kitchen
at night in New Orleans
Where sound is sautéed

on romping trombones
and throbbing bass
Where drum sticks drizzle
symbals sizzle
and rattling snares quake
It's hot for no reason
Down in New Orleans.

The city sits in the hip
of the Mississippi River's
sensual switch
Her curve births life
She dances through
Savage Bayou
Where St. Malo stole freedom
while wild indigo grew
Where Yoruba spirits still cast a grisgris
while the swamp bug symphony
strikes a syncopated beat
Where rigid time
melts
into Jazz
when melodies
get peppered
with pizzazz
Down in New Orleans.

Catacombs rise
and lift crosses to the sky
sinking in sin drenched soil
Below sea level
six feet above the devil
where the gumbo is slow to boil

Hot sauce runs thick
rich as mixed blood
with the funky sweet scent
of magnolia buds
Patois people
in kinship so close
that only last names sing secrets untold
Afro Euro Creole flavors
curry favor
in Congo Square
Down in New Orleans.

We Celebrate
Where poor boys can eat, drink, and pray
in the jambalaya jumble before Fat Tuesday
when the marching bands rumble
and the flambeaus sway
Where ancient oaks toast to hurricanes past
Where wrought iron curls
and rain stains the glass
At a Super Sunday Second Line
You can buckjump out of your mind
Party till the sun shines
and pass a real good time
down in New Orleans.

Welcome your self
out of your self
and into the taste of this town
Lose yourself
till your soul is found
Down in New Orleans.

MICHAEL MOLINA

Cajun-Spiced Tempeh Po' Boys (undressed)

PREPARATION TIME: 15 minutes
COOKING TIME: 1 hour and 45 minutes

1 pound (two 8-ounce packages) tempeh,
sliced horizontally into ½-inch fingers
½ cup extra-virgin olive oil, plus more as needed
1 large yellow onion, thinly sliced
1 teaspoon onion powder
2 teaspoons garlic powder
1 teaspoon paprika
1 teaspoon chili powder
½ teaspoon red chile flakes
¼ teaspoon cayenne pepper
1 teaspoon dried thyme
1 teaspoon dried oregano
Coarse sea salt
Freshly ground black pepper
2 large green bell peppers, cored, ribs and seeds removed,
and cut into long strips (¼ inch wide)
¼ cup tomato paste
1 tablespoon pure maple syrup
1 teaspoon balsamic vinegar
One 14.5-ounce can diced tomatoes
2 whole-wheat baguettes

- In a large bowl combine the tempeh fingers with 2 tablespoons of the olive oil and toss well.
- Warm 4 tablespoons of the olive oil in a large skillet over medium-high heat. Add the tempeh fingers and cook for 5 to 7 minutes, adding more oil if necessary, un-

til lightly browned. Turn the fingers over and cook for 5 to 7 minutes more, until lightly browned on the other side. Transfer the tempeh to a large plate lined with paper towels.

- Combine 2 tablespoons of the olive oil with the onion, onion powder, garlic powder, paprika, chili powder, red chile flakes, cayenne, thyme, oregano, 1 teaspoon salt, and 1 teaspoon black pepper in a large nonstick skillet over medium-low heat. Slowly sauté for 15 minutes, stirring often to prevent burning, until well caramelized.

- Preheat the oven to 350°F.

- Add the green bell peppers, and more oil if needed, and sauté for 10 more minutes, or until the bell peppers are softened.

- In a large bowl combine 2 cups water, the tomato paste, maple syrup, vinegar, and 2 teaspoons salt. Whisk well. Add the canned tomatoes with their juices and the onion–green pepper mixture. Stir well.

- Place the tempeh in a large casserole dish. Pour the sauce on top, covering all the tempeh fingers.

- Cover the dish with foil and bake for 1 hour, or until most of the sauce is absorbed.

- Cut each baguette in half widthwise and then slice each half lengthwise, like you would for a sandwich. Place about 5 tempeh fingers on one slice, making sure you cover it with plenty of sauce, and place another slice on top.

NOT-SO-OBVIOUS KITCHEN GEAR #5: COFFEE/SPICE GRINDER

If you're a coffee drinker, grinding your beans and making your own coffee will cut the expense of your morning java addiction. It's also a great tool for grinding spices and seeds. If you do use your grinder for coffee, get a second one for your spices and seeds.

Fresh Herb–Baked French Fries
with Creole Mustard

■■■

PREPARATION TIME: 5 minutes
INACTIVE PREPARATION TIME: At least 1 hour, or overnight
COOKING TIME: 40 minutes

We don't usually promote products, but I could never make Creole mustard better than Maison Louisianne's Creole Mustard. If it's not sold in your area you can order it at www.shutmymouth.com.

4 large russet potatoes (about 2 pounds), scrubbed
2 tablespoons extra-virgin olive oil
1 tablespoon minced fresh parsley
1 tablespoon minced fresh sage
1 tablespoon minced fresh rosemary
1 tablespoon minced fresh thyme
½ teaspoon chili powder
Coarse sea salt
Creole mustard, for serving

- Cut the potatoes into slices about ½ inch thick, then cut them ½ inch thick lengthwise into the shape of fries.
- In a large bowl, cover the potatoes with cold water, cover the bowl, and refrigerate for at least 1 hour, or overnight.
- Preheat the oven to 400°F. Line a baking sheet with parchment paper.
- Thoroughly drain the potatoes in a colander. Pat them well with paper towels until completely dry.
- In a large bowl, gently toss the potatoes with the olive oil, herbs, chili powder, and 1 teaspoon sea salt. Transfer the potatoes to the prepared pan.

- Bake for 40 minutes, gently turning a few times, until cooked thoroughly and lightly browned.
- Drain the fries on paper towels to remove any excess oil.
- Sprinkle with a little salt, if desired, and serve with Creole mustard.

Carrot Coleslaw

PREPARATION TIME: 10 minutes

INACTIVE PREPARATION TIME: At least 1 hour, or overnight

½ small green cabbage head, cored and thinly sliced

2 large carrots, grated

½ teaspoon whole-grain Dijon mustard or Creole mustard
(see Headnote, page 230)

¼ cup apple cider vinegar

1 teaspoon organic raw cane sugar

Coarse sea salt

3 tablespoons extra-virgin olive oil

2 tablespoon sesame seeds, toasted

- In a large bowl, combine the cabbage and carrots.
- In a medium bowl, combine the mustard, vinegar, sugar, and 1 teaspoon salt. Slowly add the olive oil, whisking.
- Add the dressing to the cabbage and carrots and massage well for 3 to 5 minutes. Refrigerate the slaw for at least 1 hour or overnight. Remove the slaw at least 15 minutes before serving and sprinkle with the sesame seeds.

Frozen Blackberry Slurricane

■■■

PREPARATION TIME: 5 minutes

YIELD: 2 servings (see Note)

I added my personal touch to the Hurricane, the official drink of Mardi Gras in New Orleans. After two of these you might start doing the "second line," an African-American expressive approach to funeral processions and parades in New Orleans in which celebrants dance exuberantly in the streets.

¼ cup dark rum

¼ cup light rum

½ cup passion fruit juice

¼ cup orange-pineapple-banana juice

¼ cup fresh lemon juice

½ cup frozen blackberries

3 tablespoons pure maple syrup

8 to 10 ice cubes

■ In a blender, combine all the ingredients and blend until smooth.

Note: This recipe is written for two servings, as a blender can only fit so much liquid. Make sure you have plenty of ingredients on hand so you can keep the drinks flowing.

▤ TIPS FOR PREPARING THIS MENU ▤

■ Check your calendar to see what date Mardi Gras falls on. Get some beads, cups, and a King's Cake for the celebration.

■ Soak the potatoes overnight.

■ Make the slaw and refrigerate overnight.

■ Before your guests arrive, make a few batches of Slurricanes, pour them into a pitcher, and put it in the freezer. Stir often and take the pitcher out soon before your guests arrive.

Valentine's Day Decadence

■ ■ ■

Peppered Edamame

■

Hot and Sour Shiitake Mushroom Soup

■

Sensual Vegetable Stir-Fry

■

Forbidden Black Rice

■

Chocolate-Rosemary Pudding with
Dark Chocolate–Covered Espresso Beans

■ ■ ■

Soundtrack
(provided by Suheir Hammad)

Anita Baker, *Rapture*
John Coltrane, *Coltrane for Lovers*
Abdel Halim Hafez, *Ahwak*
Maxwell, *Maxwell MTV Unplugged*
The Horace Silver Quartet, *Song for My Father*

■ ■ ■

This menu is for a two-person dinner party. The idea for the menu came from my honey,
Bethanie.

WELCOME

my generosity is not steaming
on the table and waiting
for you before you
even know you want it

come to my house friend you
will find my offering still simmering
i have not yet figured out what
you need and your tastes are mystery
still to me

i will wait for you to enter
my kitchen and once here
you can let me know what you like
sweet and slow
pepper and stirred

then we can share in this gift together
both of us giving
both of us receiving
open handed
open hearted

SUHEIR HAMMAD

Peppered Edamame

■■■

PREPARATION TIME: 5 minutes
COOKING TIME: 5 minutes

These bright green soybeans add some protein to this meal. You can find them frozen in Asian markets and health food stores. Open the pod and feed them to your lover (and vice versa).

Coarse sea salt
½ pound frozen edamame in the pod
Pinch of cayenne pepper, or to taste
Freshly ground black pepper

■ Combine 5 cups water with ½ teaspoon salt in a large pot over high heat and bring to a boil. Add the edamame and return to a boil. Cover and cook for 3 minutes. Drain in a colander.

■ In a large bowl, combine the cayenne, ¼ teaspoon black pepper, and ½ teaspoon salt. Add the edamame and toss well.

■ Serve warm in a large bowl, and place a smaller bowl on the table for discarding the pods.

Hot and Sour Shiitake Mushroom Soup

■■■

PREPARATION TIME: 10 minutes
COOKING TIME: 12 minutes

2 tablespoons arrowroot
1 tablespoon tamari
1 tablespoon rice vinegar

1 tablespoon fresh lime juice

Freshly ground white pepper

1 tablespoon extra-virgin olive oil

½ serrano chile, seeded and finely chopped

1 cup thinly sliced shiitake mushrooms

3 cups vegetable stock

½ tablespoon toasted sesame oil, for drizzling

- In a small bowl combine the arrowroot with 3 tablespoons cold water and mix well until the arrowroot is dissolved. Add the tamari, rice vinegar, lime juice, and ½ teaspoon white pepper. Mix well and set aside.
- Warm the olive oil in a medium pot over medium heat. Add the chile and mushrooms and sauté for 3 minutes, stirring well, until softened.
- Add the vegetable stock, raise the heat, and bring to a boil. Reduce the heat and simmer for 7 minutes.
- Add the arrowroot mixture to the soup, stirring constantly, until thickened, about 2 minutes. Remove from the heat.
- Ladle the soup into two bowls, drizzle each serving with sesame oil, and serve immediately.

Sensual Vegetable Stir-Fry

PREPARATION TIME: 15 minutes

COOKING TIME: 10 minutes

Apparently, the vegetables in this dish stimulate multiple appetites.

2 teaspoons arrowroot

½ cup cold apple juice

1 tablespoon apple cider vinegar

2 tablespoons tamari or shoyu

1 tablespoon minced fresh ginger

2 garlic cloves, minced

2 tablespoons sesame oil

¾ cup thinly sliced red onions

1 fresh red chile, seeded and cut in thin strips

2 large carrots, thinly sliced on the diagonal

2 ½ cups thinly sliced red cabbage (about ¼ head)

1 to 2 bunches baby bok choy, cut into bite-size pieces (to equal 2 cups)

¼ cup pine nuts

- In a small bowl, combine the arrowroot with 2 tablespoons of the apple juice and mix well until the arrowroot is completely dissolved. Add the remaining apple juice, the vinegar, tamari, ginger, and garlic. Mix well and set aside.
- Heat a large skillet or wok over high heat. Add the sesame oil and heat for 30 seconds, or until very hot but not smoking. Add the onions and the chile and stir-fry for about 2 minutes, until they start to soften. Add the carrots and stir-fry for about 2 minutes, until they start to soften. Add the cabbage and stir-fry for about 2 minutes, until the cabbage starts to soften. Add the bok choy and stir until the leaves start to wilt, about 30 seconds. Add the pine nuts and apple juice mixture, stir well, and simmer for 1 minute, until slightly thickened. Serve immediately, with Forbidden Black Rice.

Forbidden Black Rice

PREPARATION TIME: 5 minutes

INACTIVE PREPARATION TIME: At least 6 hours, or overnight

COOKING TIME: 40 minutes

Black rice has a fragrant aroma, pleasant texture, and unforgettable nutty taste. It was considered an aphrodisiac only to be enjoyed by ancient Chinese emperors and their close ones, and forbidden to commoners. You can find it at Asian grocery stores and many health food stores.

½ cup forbidden black rice

Coarse sea salt

- In a medium bowl, combine the black rice, ⅛ teaspoon salt, and ¾ cup plus 2 tablespoons water. Swish around, cover, and refrigerate at least 6 hours, or overnight.
- Place the soaked rice, water and all, in a medium saucepan over high heat and bring to a boil. Reduce the heat to low, cover, and cook for 30 minutes, or until the rice is tender but still al dente and most of the water has been absorbed.
- Remove from the heat and set aside to steam with the cover on for 10 minutes, then fluff with a fork before serving.

Chocolate-Rosemary Pudding with Dark Chocolate–Covered Espresso Beans

PREPARATION TIME: 5 minutes

INACTIVE PREPARATION TIME: At least 2 hours, or overnight

COOKING TIME: 15 minutes

If you imagine that chocolate and rosemary are a bizarre combination, you won't feel that way after experiencing this ambrosial treat. I know it doesn't quite flow with the East Asian motif of this menu, but this dessert is so decadent that I couldn't resist.

1 cup coconut milk, fresh (see page 252) or canned

3 tablespoons chopped fresh rosemary

½ cup pure maple syrup

1 teaspoon pure vanilla extract

¼ cup unsweetened cocoa powder

Fine sea salt

*1 box (¾ pound) Mori Nu firm silken tofu (this dessert only works with
    this brand because of its particular texture)*

¼ cup dark chocolate–covered espresso beans (about 24 espresso beans)
   (or dark chocolate–covered almonds)
Organic rose petals, for garnish

- Combine the coconut milk and rosemary in a small saucepan over high heat. Bring to a boil, then reduce the heat to medium-high and boil for 10 minutes, stirring often. Remove from the heat and strain into a small bowl.
- Combine 3 tablespoons of the rosemary–coconut milk mixture (reserve the rest for use in another dish such as coconut rice or coconut quinoa), with the maple syrup, vanilla, cocoa powder, and ⅛ teaspoon salt in a medium saucepan. Whisk to incorporate the cocoa powder. Bring to a boil over high heat, then reduce the heat to low and simmer for 1 minute, whisking constantly. Remove from the heat.
- Pour the mixture into a blender, add the tofu, and blend until smooth. Transfer to a medium bowl, add the espresso beans, and stir well.
- Cover with plastic and refrigerate to set for at least 2 hours, or overnight, before serving.
- Serve chilled in two small bowls placed on a plate surrounded by a bed of rose petals.

Note: This dessert can be stretched out over a few days, but you and your lover will probably eat it all that night.

▓ TIPS FOR PREPARING THIS MENU ▓

- Prepare each dish thoughtfully and lovingly with the intention of seducing your lover (or potential lover).
- Prep all the vegetables for the stir-fry a few hours ahead of time.
- Soak the rice in the refrigerator overnight.
- Make the pudding and refrigerate overnight.
- Buy organic roses to garnish the pudding and spread throughout the house.
- Create a sexy mood by lighting the room with candles, playing soft music, and lookin' fine.
- In a seductive voice, read Suheir Hammad's "Welcome" to your sweetie.
- Nibble on the edamame for a starter. Then serve the soup, and follow it with the stir-fry and black rice. And after you finish the pudding, it's on . . .

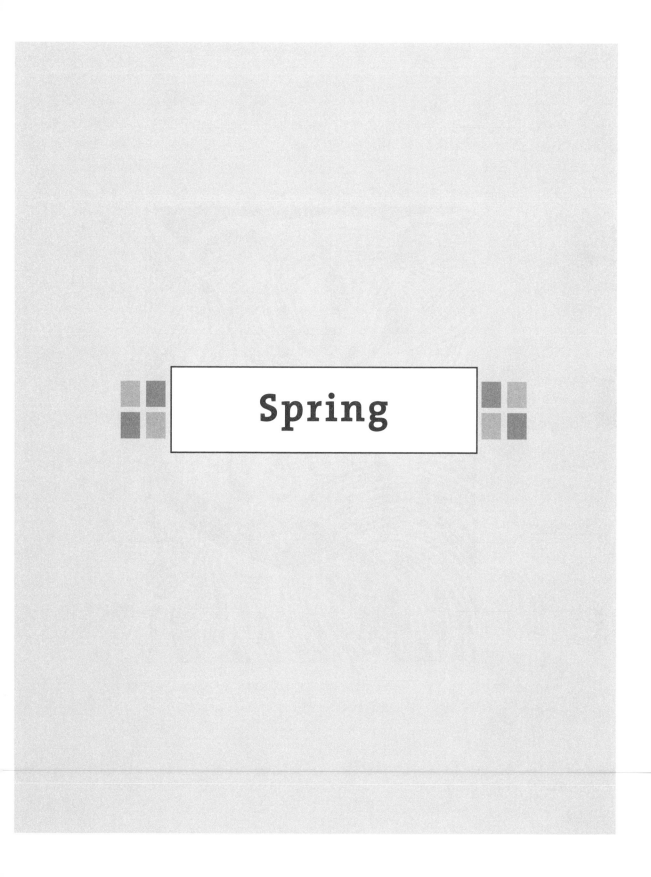

Spring

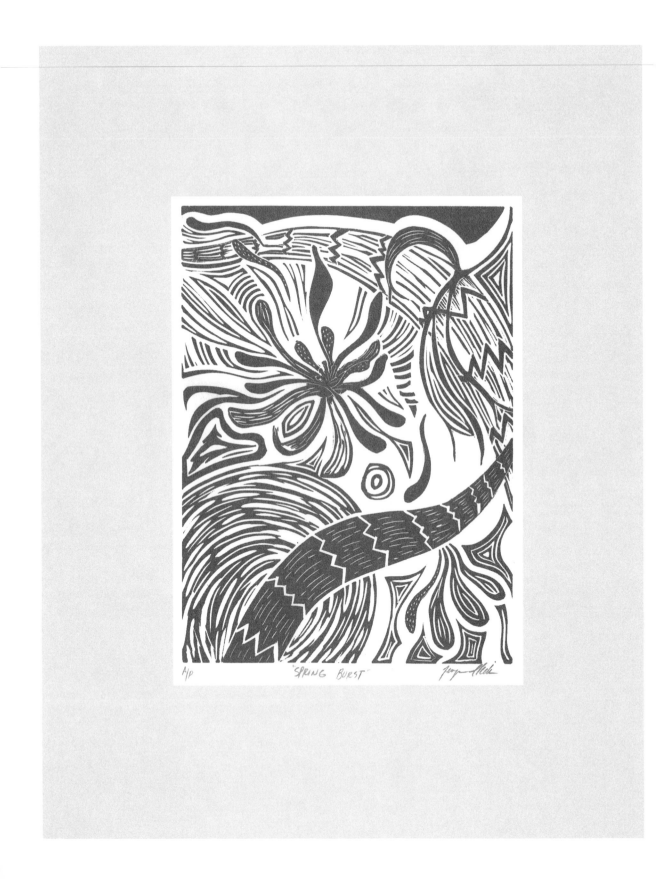

A/P   "SPRING BURST"

Lara's Cuban Comfort Meal

Both the menu and the soundtrack were provided by Lara Comstock Oramas.

■ ■ ■

Yucca Chowder

■

Watercress and Grilled Pineapple Salad with
Avocado and Sour Orange Dressing

■

Picadillo-Stuffed Chayote with Rutabaga-Garlic Sauce

■

Tropical Corn Dumplings with Maple Syrup and
Star Anise

■ ■ ■

Soundtrack

Joan Armatrading, *Joan Armatrading*
Celia Cruz, *La Reina Del R'tmo Cubano*
Richie Delamore, *More of Delamore*
The Kinks, *Kinda Kinks*
Trios de mi Cuba, *16 Grandes Exitos*

■ ■ ■

Just a taste of oregano or the feel of soft raisins in a savory mix brings me back to comfort and home. But Cuban food is so flaming meat-heavy, I was missing out on a lot of the good stuff by having given up calling our four-legged friends "dinner." This is a four-course Cuban-inspired vegan, gourmet meal (with New England flair) even my family would eat.

LARA COMSTOCK ORAMAS

Yucca Chowder

■■■

PREPARATION TIME: 15 minutes

COOKING TIME: 1 hour and 15 minutes (35 minutes if you're using store-bought stock)

The secret ingredient in this hearty chowder is recao, a more flavorful version of cilantro. It can be found in many Latino or Chinese markets and is also known as culantro, ngo-kai, or long coriander. Big up to Tía Sara, my inspiration for this and so many other wonderful things in my life.

STOCK

1 small onion

1 medium carrot

A handful of celery tops

1 teaspoon black peppercorns

3 garlic cloves, peeled

2 oregano sprigs (or 1 teaspoon dried oregano)

3 thyme sprigs (or 1 teaspoon dried thyme)

One 3-inch piece kombu

SOUP

Coarse sea salt

1 small yucca (about 10 ounces), peeled, core removed,
    and cut into ¾-inch dice

2 tablespoons extra-virgin olive oil

1 small onion, diced

¾ teaspoon ground cumin

Freshly ground black pepper

¼ cup roughly chopped tomato

4 garlic cloves, minced

1 tablespoon chopped fresh oregano (or 1 teaspoon dried)

Pinch of saffron threads, soaked in ½ cup warm water for 10 minutes

8 pieces fresh okra

1 cup fresh or frozen corn kernels

Chopped recao or cilantro, for garnish

1 lime, quartered

FOR THE STOCK

- Trim and chop the onion. Chop the carrot. Combine the onion, carrot, celery tops, peppercorns, garlic, oregano, thyme, and kombu in a 3-quart saucepan with 5 cups water. Bring to a boil over high heat, then reduce the heat to medium-low and simmer, partially covered, for 45 minutes. Remove from the heat and cool to room temperature.

FOR THE SOUP

- While the stock is simmering, combine 3 cups water with 2 teaspoons salt in a medium saucepan. Bring to a boil over high heat. Add the yucca and reduce the heat to medium. Cook the yucca for 10 minutes, or until it is almost cooked through to the center. Drain and set aside.
- Warm the olive oil in a medium saucepan over low heat. Add the onion, a pinch of salt, the cumin, ½ teaspoon black pepper, and the tomato and sauté for 10 minutes. Add the garlic and oregano and sauté another 10 minutes. This is the sofrito (see Notes).
- Strain the stock into the sofrito, and press the stock ingredients to extract all of the liquid. Add the saffron water. Raise the heat and bring the soup to a boil.
- Add the yucca, okra, and corn and bring back to a boil. Lower the heat and simmer, partially covered, for 15 minutes, or until the okra is soft but not mushy.
- Serve garnished with a sprinkle of chopped recao and a lime wedge.

Notes: You can substitute 3½ cups store-bought vegetable stock for the recipe here.

Sofrito is the flavor base of many savory Caribbean, Latin American, and Spanish dishes and consists of onions, garlic, peppers, tomatoes, and other ingredients depending on the region—all sautéed in olive oil.

Watercress and Grilled Pineapple Salad
with Avocado and Sour Orange Dressing

■■■

PREPARATION TIME: 15 minutes
COOKING TIME: 8 minutes

Watercress is peppery, delicious, and full of beta-carotene, calcium, and tons of other vitamins and minerals. It, like many other vegetables in Cuba, was cultivated by the island's large Chinese population.

SALAD

½ cup pepitas

1 large bunch of watercress, trimmed

¾ cup chopped pineapple, grilled and cooled

1 small carrot, shredded

DRESSING

½ Hass avocado

Juice of 2 sour oranges, or juice of 1 orange and 1 lime (to make ½ cup)

2 teaspoons pure maple syrup

3 tablespoons extra-virgin olive oil

1 small garlic clove

Coarse sea salt

Freshly ground black pepper

FOR THE SALAD

- Preheat a cast-iron skillet over high heat. When it's hot, throw in the pepitas and roast, moving them continuously for about 2 minutes, or until the seeds are just beginning to brown. Remove from the pan and set aside to cool to room temperature.
- Combine the watercress, pineapple, and carrot in a large bowl.

- Combine the avocado, citrus juice, maple syrup, olive oil, garlic, ½ teaspoon salt, and black pepper to taste in a blender or food processor and blend until smooth. With the motor running, add ¼ cup cold water in a thin stream until the dressing reaches your desired consistency, then stop. Open the top and taste the dressing. Adjust the seasonings.
- To serve, toss the salad and divide into 4 servings. Pour on the dressing and sprinkle the pepitas over each serving. Leftover dressing may be refrigerated for up to 5 days.

Picadillo-Stuffed Chayote with Rutabaga-Garlic Sauce

PREPARATION TIME: 30 minutes
COOKING TIME: 1 hour and 30 minutes

The raisins in the picadillo provide the perfect sweet balance to a lot of complex flavors.

CHAYOTE
4 medium chayote, cut in half
1 tablespoon extra-virgin olive oil
Coarse sea salt
Freshly ground black pepper

SAUCE
2 tablespoons extra-virgin olive oil
2 onions, diced large
8 garlic cloves, minced
Pinch of nutmeg
¼ teaspoon ground cumin

Coarse sea salt

Freshly ground white pepper

1 cup chopped rutabaga

¾ cup cooked chayote (see Directions)

¼ cup walnuts, lightly toasted, skins rubbed off

PICADILLO

1 russet or other baking potato, scrubbed and diced medium

2 tablespoons plus 2 teaspoons extra-virgin olive oil

2 small onions, diced small

½ cup finely diced green bell pepper

5 shiitake mushroom caps, chopped small

Coarse sea salt

Freshly ground black pepper

¼ teaspoon ground cumin

4 garlic cloves, minced

1 tablespoon chopped fresh rosemary (or 1 teaspoon dried)

1 teaspoon fresh thyme (or ½ teaspoon dried)

2 tablespoons capers, drained

2 tablespoons chopped green olives

1 small tomato, seeded and chopped

½ cup raisins

3 tablespoons apple cider vinegar

One 8-ounce package tempeh, crumbled

¼ cup pepitas, toasted and roughly chopped

½ cup pistachios, shelled, toasted, and roughly chopped

¼ cup roughly chopped flat-leaf parsley

*1 green plantain, sliced very thin into 2-inch strips and
fried quickly in hot oil*

FOR THE CHAYOTE

- Preheat the oven to 350°F. Line a baking sheet with parchment paper.
- Lightly coat the chayote halves with the olive oil, and sprinkle with 1 teaspoon salt

and ½ teaspoon black pepper. Lay the halves face down on the prepared baking sheet. Roast on the middle rack of the oven for 50 minutes, or until a knife easily pierces the flesh of the chayote (turn the chayote right-side-up when testing). Set aside to cool, then scoop out the flesh and save it.

- While you're roasting the chayotes, coat the potato for the picadillo in 2 teaspoons of the olive oil and a pinch of salt. Spread the pieces on a parchment-lined baking sheet. Roast in the same oven as the chayote halves for 20 minutes, stirring once, until the pieces are nicely golden. Set aside. Keep the oven on.

FOR THE SAUCE

- Warm the olive oil in a medium saucepan over medium heat. Add the onions, reduce the heat to low, and sweat the onions for 10 minutes, or until they are translucent. Add the garlic, nutmeg, cumin, 1 teaspoon salt, and a pinch of white pepper. Sauté for another 10 minutes, stirring occasionally.
- Add the rutabaga, chayote flesh, and 2½ cups water. Raise the heat to high and bring to a boil. Lower the heat to low, cover, and cook for 20 to 25 minutes, or until the rutabaga is soft when pierced with a fork.
- Transfer half of the mixture to a blender or food processor, along with half of the walnuts, and blend for 30 seconds, or until the sauce is smooth and free of lumps. Pour the sauce into a casserole dish large enough to hold 8 chayote halves. Repeat with the second half of the sauce and set aside.

FOR THE PICADILLO

- Make the picadillo while you're making the sauce. Warm the remaining 2 tablespoons olive oil in a large skillet over low heat. Add the onions, bell pepper, and mushrooms. Turn the heat to medium and sauté for 10 minutes, or until the onions are translucent.
- Add 1 teaspoon salt, ¼ teaspoon black pepper, the cumin, garlic, rosemary, and thyme and sauté for 3 more minutes.
- Add the capers, olives, tomatoes, raisins, vinegar, tempeh, and water to just cover the tempeh. Raise the heat to high and bring to a boil. Reduce the heat to low and cook for 15 minutes, stirring once halfway through. Add the roasted potatoes, pepitas, and pistachios, stir again, and cook for another 5 to 10 minutes, until all

the liquid is evaporated and the tempeh has begun to brown. Taste and adjust the seasoning.

To assemble

- Place the scooped-out chayote halves face-up in the sauce-filled casserole dish. Scoop about ¼ cup of picadillo filling into each chayote half and pack firmly. The chayote shells should be brimming over. Bake for about 15 minutes, or until the top of the picadillo has begun to brown and the sauce is very hot.
- Serve hot, 2 halves per person, with sauce spooned on top and sprinkled with parsley and plantain sticks.

Tropical Corn Dumplings with Maple Syrup and Star Anise

PREPARATION TIME: 10 minutes
COOKING TIME: 20 to 23 minutes

This dish can be thrown together at the last minute. I've also made it with pineapple, strawberries, and rhubarb, but you can use any local or seasonal fruit. This is a variation on an old New England "slump" or "grunt."

¼ cup coconut milk, fresh (see page 252) or canned

1 teaspoon apple cider vinegar, white vinegar, or lemon juice

¼ cup fresh or frozen sweet corn kernels

1 tablespoon safflower or canola oil

¾ cup diced fresh mango (preferably Haitian) or guava pulp, seeds removed

¾ cup grade-B maple syrup

3 whole star anise

½ cup whole-wheat pastry or whole-spelt flour

¼ cup fine cornmeal

½ teaspoon baking powder

¼ teaspoon baking soda

½ teaspoon ground cinnamon

Fine sea salt

¼ cup fresh shredded or dried coconut

½ cup toasted and roughly chopped cashews

- In a small bowl combine the coconut milk and vinegar. Set aside for 10 minutes.
- Combine the coconut and vinegar mixture, the corn, and safflower oil in a blender or food processor. Puree for 2 minutes, until the corn has broken down to liquid.
- Place the mango, maple syrup, 2 cups water, and star anise in a small, deep, heavy-bottomed saucepan. Bring to a boil over high heat. Reduce the heat to low and simmer, covered, for 5 minutes.
- Sift the flour, cornmeal, baking powder, baking soda, cinnamon, and ¼ teaspoon salt into a medium bowl. Stir in the coconut.
- Add the liquid to the flour and stir until dough is just moistened (using your clean hands works great). The dough will be rather dry. Don't overmix or your dumplings will be tough.
- Drop 9 spoonfuls of dough into the hot maple syrup mixture. Cover and simmer over low heat until the dumplings have expanded, 15 to 18 minutes, watching that the maple syrup does not begin to scorch. Test one at 15 minutes—they're done when they look fluffy inside. Remove the star anise.
- Serve warm with sauce ladled on top and sprinkled with the cashews.

MAKING COCONUT MILK

Fresh coconut milk is easy to make and a vast improvement over the canned variety. Buy a fresh coconut, and using a hammer pound holes through the eyes with a screwdriver, drain it, and crack it open. Pry the flesh from the shell, break it up with your hands, peel off the brown skin if you're ambitious, and then process the coconut in a food processor, adding 1¾ to 2 cups very hot water while processing. Allow to sit for 10 minutes, then strain it through several layers of cheesecloth. Voilà!

Have a backup can of coconut milk in case the coconut you pick has gone bad, which can throw a wrench into an otherwise excellent evening.

TIPS FOR PREPARING THIS MENU

- This menu was designed so that most of the ingredients can be purchased at any well-stocked grocery store in a Latino area. You can also ask farmers at your local farmers' market if they would start planting yucca, chayote, and organic plantains.
- Be mindful, breathe, and invoke the spirit of your grandmother.
- Make the soup up to the point right before you add the yucca, okra, and corn a few hours ahead of time. Add the vegetables 15 minutes before serving.
- Toast the pepitas and grill the pineapple for the salad and refrigerate overnight.
- Make the avocado and sour orange salad dressing a few hours ahead of time and refrigerate it.
- The day before, roast the chayote and make the picadillo and rutabaga-garlic sauce. You can assemble the whole dish a day ahead and refrigerate it, then pop it in the oven about an hour before you're ready to serve. If you're warming it up directly from the refrigerator, cover it with foil for the first half hour.

LUDIE AND ELIZABETH'S AFRO-LATINA TAPAS

Both the menu and the soundtrack were provided by Ludie Minaya and Elizabeth Johnson.

■ ■ ■

Grandma's Pastelitos

■

Lima Bean and Corn Dumplings with Sage

■

Mofongo with Wild Mushroom Sauce

■

Black Bean Spread

■

Vegetable Salad with Balsamic Vinaigrette

■ ■ ■

Soundtrack

Break'n Bossa!—The American Chapter (Compilation)
Fertile Ground, *Spiritual War*
Simply Salsa (Compilation)
Cassandra Wilson, *Belly of the Sun*
Zap Mama, *Ancestry in Progress*

■ ■ ■

Making these tapas reflects our efforts to keep the traditional cuisine of our Southern and Latino ancestors alive, with a modern twist. We honor the ability of our foremothers and forefathers to pepper Old World dishes with New World ingredients and re-create the flavors of their homeland. They were truly the creators of the first "fusion" cuisine. These recipes continue this tradition as we make our grandmothers' recipes more modern and health-supportive. We invite you to remember *your* family recipes, preserve them, and update them if you like. Share them with your loved ones, keeping ancient rituals and foods alive.

This is a tapas dinner meant to be shared with close friends. This dinner comfortably serves four, but it can accommodate a few more people.

LUDIE MINAYA AND ELIZABETH JOHNSON

Grandma's Pastelitos

PREPARATION TIME: 30 minutes
COOKING TIME: About 1 hour and 30 minutes

Grandma usually puts chicken or beef in these dumplings. We substituted marinated tempeh for the meat. We did, however, keep Grandma's Old World spicing. We think you'll find it's just as good.

One 8-ounce package tempeh, cut into 4 pieces
1 large russet potato, peeled and cut in half
6 cups low-sodium vegetable stock
2 garlic cloves, smashed and peeled
4 tablespoons extra-virgin olive oil
1 medium onion, sliced into thin half-moons
4 garlic cloves, minced
Coarse sea salt
Freshly ground black pepper
1 teaspoon dried oregano
2 tablespoons tomato paste
¼ cup raisins, soaked in warm water to cover until plump
    (about 10 minutes)
1 tablespoon plus 1 teaspoon capers
1 package square 3½-inch wonton skins
Grapeseed or olive oil, for frying

- Combine the tempeh, potato, stock, and smashed garlic in a medium saucepan over high heat. Bring to a boil, then lower the heat and simmer for 30 minutes, or until the potato is fork-tender. Using a slotted spoon, remove the tempeh and potato from the broth and allow them to cool. Strain the cooking liquid into a small bowl and set aside. Shred the tempeh using a grater and set aside. Cut the potato into ¼-inch squares and set aside.

- Heat the olive oil in a large sauté pan over medium-low heat. Add the onions and sauté until reduced in size and browned and sweet, 20 to 30 minutes. Add the minced garlic, reserved tempeh, ½ teaspoon salt, ½ teaspoon black pepper, and oregano and cook for 5 to 10 minutes, or until the tempeh is lightly browned. Turn up the heat and stir in the tomato paste and 2 cups of the reserved cooking liquid. Cook until the liquid is absorbed, about 10 minutes.

- Remove the raisins from the soaking water. Add them to the pan, along with the capers and potatoes. Stir to combine and cook for about 2 minutes, to warm through. Taste and add more salt and pepper if needed. Set aside to cool.

- When the filling has cooled, lay out 5 wonton skins at a time on a work surface. Set up a small bowl filled with warm water. Place 1 heaping teaspoon of the filling in the middle of each wonton skin. Dip your fingers lightly into the water, then glide your fingers along the edge of each filled square. Fold one corner of each square over to the far corner, forming a triangle. Press tightly with a fork to seal. Set aside. Repeat until you've used up all the filling.

- Preheat the oven to 200°F.

- Fill a medium skillet with ½ inch grapeseed oil. Place over medium-high heat and heat the oil until it's hot. Add the pastelitos in one layer, frying until golden brown, about 30 seconds on each side. Transfer to a paper towel–lined plate to drain. If not serving right away, place the pastelitos on a baking sheet and transfer to the oven to keep warm.

Lima Bean and Corn Dumplings with Sage

■ ■ ■

PREPARATION TIME: 30 minutes
INACTIVE PREPARATION TIME: Overnight
COOKING TIME: About 1 hour

Lima beans and corn are often used in succotash in the Southern states. We made this traditional dish tapas-friendly by wrapping the dumplings in wonton skins. They are lightly crisp, sweet, and tangy.

½ pound dried lima beans
1 bay leaf
3 tablespoons extra-virgin olive oil
½ small yellow onion, finely chopped
2 ears of corn, kernels scraped off the cob
3 tablespoons chopped pine nuts
2 cloves garlic, minced
2 tablespoons minced fresh sage
1 tablespoon minced fresh thyme
⅛ teaspoon cayenne pepper
⅛ teaspoon freshly grated nutmeg
Juice of ½ lemon
½ teaspoon lemon zest
Coarse sea salt
1 package square 3½-inch wonton skins
Grapeseed or olive oil, for frying

- In medium bowl, combine the lima beans with water to cover by a few inches. Let soak overnight. Drain and rinse thoroughly.
- Place the lima beans in a medium pot. Add the bay leaf and add water to cover by 2 inches. Place over high heat and bring to a boil. Then reduce the heat and cook,

partially covered, until the lima beans are tender enough to mash easily with a fork, about 30 minutes, checking occasionally to skim any foam that rises and to remove any lima bean skins that float to the top.

- Meanwhile, heat the olive oil in a medium sauté pan over medium-low heat. Add the onion and cook, stirring, for 1 minute. Add the corn kernels and cook for 10 minutes, or until soft. Add the pine nuts and cook until fragrant and lightly browned, about 3 minutes. Add the garlic and cook 1 minute more.

- Stir in the sage, thyme, cayenne, nutmeg, lemon juice and zest, and salt to taste. Cook for 5 minutes for the flavors to combine. Set aside.

- When lima beans are cooked, remove the bay leaf and drain into a colander. Return them to the pot. Add 1 teaspoon salt. Using a potato masher or wooden or metal spoon, mash the lima beans. Add the corn mixture to the lima beans. Taste and add more salt, pepper, or lemon juice if needed. Set aside to cool.

- Preheat the oven to 200°F.

- When the filling has cooled, lay out 5 wonton skins at a time on a work surface. Set up a small bowl filled with warm water. Place 1 heaping teaspoon of the filling in the middle of each wonton skin. Dip your fingers lightly into the warm water, then glide your fingers along the edge of each filled square. Fold one corner of each square over to the far corner, forming a triangle. Seal the dumpling by using the back of a fork to press the skins together. Set aside. Repeat until all the filling is used.

- Fill a medium skillet with ½ inch grapeseed oil. Place over medium-high heat and heat the oil until it's hot. Add the dumplings in one layer, frying until golden brown, about 30 seconds on each side. Transfer to a paper towel–lined plate to drain. If not serving right away, place the dumplings on a baking sheet and transfer to the oven to keep warm.

Mofongo with Wild Mushroom Sauce

■■■

PREPARATION TIME: 15 minutes
COOKING TIME: About 1 hour

Mofongo is the national dish of Puerto Rico. It is usually made with pork, but we chose to use the earthy, rich flavors of wild mushrooms to give this dish its hearty feel. This should be the last dish you make from this menu. It is best served hot!

MUSHROOM SAUCE
5 tablespoons extra-virgin olive oil
1 medium onion, sliced into half-moons
4 garlic cloves, minced
10 ounces wild mushrooms, such as shiitake, Baby Bella,
      or bluefoot, sliced ¼ inch thick
Coarse sea salt
Freshly ground black pepper
½ teaspoon dried oregano
1 tablespoon balsamic vinegar
¼ cup rum
1½ cups low-sodium vegetable stock
2 tablespoons all-purpose flour
1 tablespoon minced fresh oregano

MOFONGO
Olive oil, for frying
4 green plantains, peeled and cut into ¼-inch rounds
3 garlic cloves, minced
Fine sea salt

FOR THE MUSHROOM SAUCE

- Heat the olive oil in a large sauté pan over medium-low heat. Add the onion and sauté, stirring occasionally, until reduced in size, browned, and sweet, 25 to 30 minutes.
- Add the garlic and cook until fragrant but not browned, about 1½ minutes. Add the mushrooms, ½ teaspoon salt, ½ teaspoon black pepper, and the dried oregano. Raise the heat to medium and sauté until the mushrooms are nicely browned, about 5 minutes.
- Add the rum, stirring, removing any bits from the bottom of the pan. Cook for 5 minutes, or until the mushrooms have absorbed most of the liquid. Add the stock, bring to a boil, then lower the heat to a simmer.
- Meanwhile, in a small cup or bowl, combine the flour with 4 tablespoons water and stir until dissolved. Pour the flour mixture into the pan and stir to combine. Cook another 5 minutes, or until the sauce is thickened. Sprinkle with the fresh oregano. Set aside.

FOR THE MOFONGO

- Heat the olive oil in a large sauté pan over medium-high heat. Add some of the plantains in one layer. Fry until barely golden, about 3 minutes each side. Using a slotted spoon, remove the plantains from the heat and place on a paper towel–lined plate to drain. Let the oil get hot before adding more plantains, and add more oil if necessary as you go along.
- In a medium bowl, while the plantains are still hot, using a potato masher or the bottom of a cup, mash the plantains with some of the garlic and a pinch of salt. Repeat until all the plantains are fried and mashed.
- Serve the mofongo on individual plates, each shaped into a small volcano. Top with the mushroom sauce.

Black Bean Spread

PREPARATION TIME: 10 minutes
INACTIVE PREPARATION TIME: Overnight
COOKING TIME: 30 minutes

½ pound dried black beans
1 bay leaf
1 tablespoon ground cumin
1 teaspoon ground coriander
⅛ teaspoon cayenne pepper
1 garlic clove
4 tablespoons chopped fresh cilantro
¼ cup fresh lemon juice
3 tablespoons raw tahini
6 tablespoons extra-virgin olive oil
½ teaspoon coarse sea salt

- Place the beans in a medium bowl and add water to cover. Let soak overnight. Drain and rinse well.
- Place the beans in a medium pot. Add the bay leaf and water to cover by 2 inches. Place over high heat and bring to a boil. Then reduce the heat and cook, partially covered, for about 30 minutes, or until the beans are fork-tender. Drain, reserving 1 cup of the cooking liquid. Allow the beans to cool.
- In a food processor, combine the beans with the remaining ingredients and process until smooth. With the motor running, add ¼ cup of the reserved cooking liquid, adding more if needed. Taste and add more salt and lemon juice if needed. Serve with pita bread or tortilla chips.

Vegetable Salad with Balsamic Vinaigrette

■■■

PREPARATION TIME: 20 minutes

The dressing is especially good with late spring or summer vegetables and lettuce. Remember to toss your greens with a little salt and pepper before dressing them.

SALAD

½ pound mesclun

1 small cucumber, peeled and cut into ¼-inch thick half-moons

½ pint cherry tomatoes

1 bunch asparagus, stems peeled and cut on the bias into ½-inch pieces

2 red, yellow, or orange peppers, cored, seeded, and cut into thin slices

1 mango, cut into medium dice (optional)

Fine sea salt

DRESSING

½ cup best-quality balsamic vinegar

½ teaspoon minced red onion

1 tablespoon plus 1 teaspoon organic raw cane sugar

1 tablespoon minced fresh cilantro

1 teaspoon fine sea salt

¼ teaspoon freshly ground black pepper

¼ cup best-quality extra-virgin olive oil

- In a large bowl combine all the salad ingredients.
- Sprinkle lightly with salt and toss to combine. Set aside.
- In a medium bowl combine all dressing ingredients except the olive oil. Stir until the sugar dissolves. Add the oil in a slow, steady stream, whisking, until emulsified. Toss the salad with ¼ cup of the dressing. Add more dressing if needed. The remaining dressing can be used for another salad. This will last up to one week, refrigerated.

▌ TIPS FOR PREPARING THIS MENU ▐

The day before:
- Soak all the beans.
- Prepare the dressing for the salad.

A few hours before:
- Prepare the dumpling and pastelito fillings.
- Make the mushroom sauce.
- Prepare the plantains for the mofongo, placing them in salted water until you're ready to fry them (make sure you dry them thoroughly before frying).
- Make the black bean spread.
- Combine the salad ingredients in a large bowl and cover with a damp paper towel (do not dress the salad).

At dinner:
- Set out the black bean spread with chips and pita so you'll have something to eat right away.
- As a part of the dinner, invite your friends into the kitchen to make their own dumplings and pastelitos and to help make the mofongo. Traditionally, the kitchen has been the hub of activity at home—gathering around the hearth gets everyone together, talking and putting energy into the food. It develops a sense of community and breaks the ice. It also takes a load off of you!

Simply Macrobiotic

■ ■ ■

Miso Soup with Button Mushrooms

■

Brown Basmati Rice Pilaf with French Lentils

■

Teriyaki Tofu Triangles

■

Pickled Carrots

■

Roasted Brown Rice Tea

■ ■ ■

Soundtrack

(provided by Peter Berley)

Bela Fleck, *Drive*
Billie Holiday and Lester Young, *A Musical Romance*
Keith Jarrett, *The Köln Concert*
Talking Heads, *Stop Making Sense*
Lennie Tristano, *Lennie Tristano / New Tristano*

■ ■ ■

I, along with several of my friends, used to make fun of macrobiotics and anything resembling it. We would always ridicule any meals that included brown rice and roasted vegetables. ("That's so seventies," we would say.) But after hearing several stories about macrobiotics helping reverse cancers, I decided to do more research into this hippie diet. I soon discovered that macrobiotics is so much more than a diet—it's a philosophy of living in harmony with one's environment. The diet is less dogmatic than I thought, too—one's individual tastes, needs, work, environment, and the like should all be taken into consideration.

Here I have created some tasty macrobiotic dishes that might inspire you to explore this lifestyle more. The flavors in this menu are mild and the recipes are a nice change for folks used to eating rich foods.

Miso Soup with Button Mushrooms

■ ■ ■

PREPARATION TIME: 10 minutes
INACTIVE PREPARATION TIME: 20 minutes
COOKING TIME: 35 minutes

Miso soup is often the first course in macrobiotic meals.

One 3-inch piece wakame
2 cups chopped dandelion greens
1 large carrot, coarsely grated
½ cup button mushrooms, stems removed and thinly sliced
¼ cup dark barley (mugi) miso
1 scallion, trimmed and thinly sliced

- In a medium saucepan, soak the wakame in 6 cups water for 20 minutes, or until softened. Remove the wakame from the water. Chop the wakame into bite-size pieces and set aside.
- Bring the soaking water to a boil over high heat. Add the dandelions, reduce the heat to low, cover, and simmer for 20 minutes, or until softened.
- Add the carrot, mushrooms, and wakame and simmer, covered, for 10 minutes.
- Pour ¼ cup of the broth into a small bowl. Add the miso and stir to dissolve. Add this mixture to the pot and simmer for 2 more minutes (do not boil, as you will destroy the miso's vitality). Taste and add more miso to intensify the flavor if desired.
- Serve immediately, garnished with the scallions.

Brown Basmati Rice Pilaf
with French Lentils

■ ■ ■

PREPARATION TIME: 5 minutes
INACTIVE PREPARATION TIME: Overnight
COOKING TIME: 1 hour and 15 minutes

In macrobiotic diets, eating whole grains is extremely important. In fact, at least half the total volume of a meal should be whole grains. While most people associate macrobiotics with brown rice, many other grains, such as millet, whole oats, amaranth, quinoa, spelt, and noodles (udon, soba, rice, whole-wheat) can be included in this diet. Here brown basmati rice is a nice change from short- or medium-grain brown rice.

1 cup brown basmati rice
3 tablespoons shoyu or tamari
1 tablespoon extra-virgin olive oil
¼ cup French lentils (or brown lentils), sorted, soaked, and rinsed

- In a medium bowl, combine the brown rice, 1 tablespoon of the shoyu, and 2¼ cups water. Swish around, cover, and refrigerate overnight. Drain.
- Warm the olive oil in a medium saucepan over medium heat. Add the rice and sauté for 4 minutes, stirring well with a wooden spoon. Add the remaining 2 tablespoons shoyu and sauté for 1 additional minute, stirring often with a wooden spoon. Add 2 cups water and bring to a boil. Cover, reduce the heat to low, and cook for 20 minutes. Stir in the lentils and cover again. Cook for an additional 40 minutes.
- Remove from heat and steam with cover on for at least 10 minutes before serving.

Teriyaki Tofu Triangles

PREPARATION TIME: 10 minutes
COOKING TIME: 1 hour and 10 minutes

2 pounds extra-firm tofu (2 large tofu cakes), frozen, thawed,
*   and pressed (see Box, page 267)*
About ¼ cup extra-virgin olive oil,
*   plus more for frying*
½ cup shoyu
2 teaspoons tomato paste
¼ cup rice vinegar
½ cup apple juice
¼ cup pure maple syrup
1 tablespoon minced fresh ginger
1 garlic clove, minced

- Preheat the oven to 350°F.
- Place each tofu cake on its side and cut it into thirds. Keeping the layers together, cut the tofu diagonally, making 6 long triangles, then cut the triangles down the middle to make 12 smaller triangles. Pat each triangle well with paper towels.
- Warm 2 tablespoons of the olive oil in a large skillet over medium heat. Fry the tofu triangles in one snug layer until golden brown, 7 to 10 minutes on each side. Add more oil as needed. Drain the tofu triangles on paper towels.
- In a large bowl, combine the shoyu, tomato paste, vinegar, apple juice, maple syrup, 1 tablespoon of the olive oil, the ginger, and garlic. Whisk well.
- Arrange the tofu pieces in 2 snug layers in a baking dish. Pour the teriyaki sauce on top. Cover with aluminum foil and bake for 15 minutes. Turn over and bake for 15 more minutes.

Freezing, Pressing, and Marinating Tofu

Tofu is synonymous for many people with bland—the dangerous "b" word in health-supportive cooking. But it doesn't have to be. Here's a little tip to prevent this unfortunate fate. For many dishes, we suggest you marinate your tofu first (in a vegetable broth or thin marinade of your choice). You can do so by simmering it on the stovetop or baking it in an oven. Once the tofu is thoroughly marinated, you can bake, broil, or barbecue to your heart's content without fear of blandness.

But first you need to press it. Recipes that use firm tofu—as opposed to silken tofu, which is good for nondairy dressings and desserts—often call for it to be pressed. This procedure extracts excess water from the tofu and allows it to absorb marinades more easily. It also makes the tofu block more uniformly firm. To press a block of extra-firm tofu, wrap it in several paper towels or a clean kitchen towel, place it in a large bowl or a clean kitchen sink, and place a heavy weight on top for 1 hour, turning after 30 minutes, until most of the liquid is pressed out and absorbed by the towel.

Freezing tofu gives it a chewier texture in addition to increasing its ability to absorb marinades. Leave the tofu in its package and freeze it for at least twenty-four hours, then thaw in the refrigerator for 8 to 10 hours, or for 3 hours at room temperature. After it's thawed, drain, press, and marinate in a sauce of your choice.

Pickled Carrots

PREPARATION TIME: 10 minutes

INACTIVE PREPARATION TIME: At least 24 hours

COOKING TIME: 5 minutes

Sometimes I add spices to this recipe to jazz it up, but spices are normally avoided in macrobiotic diets, so I omit them here. If you want to lift the flavor of these pickles, combine 2 teaspoons brown mustard seeds and 1 teaspoon white peppercorns with the water, vinegar, sugar, and salt in the second step of this recipe.

2 or 3 large carrots (about 1 pound), peeled

1 cup white balsamic vinegar or apple cider vinegar
    or other clear vinegar

2 tablespoons organic raw cane sugar

Coarse sea salt

- Cut the carrots into sticks that are 2 inches long and ¼ inch thick.
- Combine 2 cups water, the vinegar, sugar, and 1 teaspoon salt in a medium saucepan over high heat. Bring to a boil and add the carrots. Bring back to a boil for 1 minute, then remove from the heat.
- Transfer the carrots and liquid to a glass container. Let cool and cover.
- Refrigerate the covered pickles for at least 24 hours before serving. (They will keep for up to 1 week in the refrigerator.)

Roasted Brown Rice Tea

■ ■ ■

PREPARATION TIME: 5 minutes
COOKING TIME: 15 minutes

I can't decide if I like to drink brown rice tea more for its nutty fragrance or its flavor.

1 cup brown rice
6 cups rice milk
3 tablespoons pure maple syrup,
plus more to taste

- Roast the rice in a large skillet over medium-high heat, stirring often with a wooden spoon to prevent from burning, until the rice is fragrant, about 3 to 5 minutes.
- Combine the rice, 6 cups water, the rice milk, and maple syrup in a medium saucepan over high heat. Bring to a boil, then reduce the heat to low and simmer, partially covered, for 15 minutes.
- Strain the tea into a pitcher and serve hot in mugs. Have some extra maple syrup on hand for your guests to sweeten their cups as they like.

▦ TIPS FOR PREPARING THIS MENU ▦

- Serve the miso soup first. Then serve the rice pilaf (which tastes great with the teriyaki sauce) and the tofu. The pickles can be served in a bowl placed on the table so guests can eat them at their leisure.
- Soak the rice up to 24 hours before cooking.
- Prepare your pickles a few days before.
- You can prepare the tea a day or two earlier and warm it up at dinner.

These suggestions are from Katrine Pollari, owner of Olivino Wines in Brooklyn, New York.

Down South of the U.S. Border (La Linea)

The juicy and bright acidity of a Torrontes from Argentina will enhance the flavors of this menu. A good choice is the Pircas Negras Torrontes, made with organic grapes from the Famatina Valley in Argentina.

Beets, Limes, and Rice: Salad Selection for Heads

For summer salads try an Italian Prosecco such as Zardetto Prosecco Brut. The fruity effervescence captures the essence of summer afternoons.

Afrodiasporic Cookout

This menu cries out for a refreshing summer white. Try Duck Walk Vineyards' Southampton White. The gentle notes of green apple, pear, and citrus linger through the soft finish.

After-Dinner Dessert Buffet

A lush, creamy Moscato, aromatically redolent of honeysuckle and ripe peach, will go well with this dessert buffet. Dolce Sogno from Borgo Maragliano is perfect.

¡Grub Latinoamericano!

The intense array of flavors in this menu calls for a wine with a hint of fruitiness to refresh the palate. A young rose Chile is just the wine. La Palma Rose from Vina la Rosa is a great bargain.

More Than One Side (Dish) to Thanksgiving

A fruity zinfandel is a marvelous companion for the variety of flavors of this meal. The organic zinfandel from Frey Vineyards in Mendocino, California, is a delicious classic choice.

New Millennium Soul Food

A light, slightly fruity Riesling will complement this meal well. Covey Run's Riesling from the Columbia Valley in Washington State is a good choice.

Mardi Gras Grub (Phat Tuesday)

A French Vouvray has just the right burst of fresh fruitiness to tame the Cajun/Creole heat of this menu. The Vouvray from Benoit Gautier in the Loire Valley is lovely.

Valentine's Day Decadence

Only a sparkling will do when one is fanning the flames of a romantic meal, and none does it better than Lou Lou, a light, heady, fruity Clairette de Die from high up in the French Alps.

Lara's Cuban Comfort Meal

A young bright, fruity Grenache will enhance, not overwhelm, this meal's flavors. Try Vina Borgia from Bodegas Borsao in Borja, Spain.

Ludie and Elizabeth's Afro-Latina Tapas

The delicate balance of a crisp, clean Johannesburg Riesling will refresh palates that have been tantalized by the multitude of flavors in this meal. Go organic with Badger Mountain's Riesling from Washington State.

RESOURCES

Ideas for Action

Danger Zone: Top Fruits and Vegetables to Buy Organic

In 2003, the Washington, D.C.–based Environmental Working Group examined more than 100,000 U.S. government pesticide test results. Their researchers found 192 different pesticides on 46 fresh fruits and vegetables, and determined that we can lower our risk of pesticide exposure by as much as 90 percent just by choosing organic varieties of the top twelve most contaminated fruits and vegetables. And they are . . . (drum roll please):

FRUIT

APPLES	NECTARINES	RED RASPBERRIES
CHERRIES	PEACHES	STRAWBERRIES
IMPORTED GRAPES	PEARS	

(*Note:* If you're using citrus zest, be sure to choose organic fruits, since pesticide residues can linger on the fruit's skin.)

VEGETABLES

BELL PEPPERS	CELERY	POTATOES	SPINACH

To download a wallet-size guide to pesticides in produce, visit foodnews.org.

Chapter-by-Chapter Resources for Action

For more resources for your community food audit, see the worksheet at the end of the book and visit us online at **eatgrub.org**.

Resources for Chapter 1: Shattering the Illusions

Fairness in Food, Farming, and Trade Policy
Action Group on Erosion, Technology, and Concentration | etcgroup.org
Promoting the conservation and sustainable advancement of cultural and ecological diversity and human rights.

Institute for Agriculture and Trade Policy | iatp.org
Promoting family farms, rural communities, and ecosystems around the world through research and education, science and technology, and advocacy.

Institute for Food and Development Policy | foodfirst.org
Highlighting root causes and solutions to global hunger and poverty and committed to establishing food as a fundamental human right. Food First was cofounded by Joseph Collins and Frances Moore Lappé and is a member-supported, nonprofit "people's" think tank and education-for-action center.

National Campaign for Sustainable Agriculture | sustainableagriculture.net
Educating the public on the importance of a sustainable food and agriculture system that is economically viable, environmentally sound, socially just, and humane. Sign up for their action alerts to keep abreast of critical policy issues.

Organization for Competitive Markets | competitivemarkets.com
Working to reinvigorate antitrust law and competition policy and reclaiming competitive markets in agriculture for farmers, ranchers, and rural communities.

Safe and Clean Food Supply

Beyond Pesticides | beyondpesticides.org

Promoting public health and the environment by identifying the risks of conventional pest management practices and promoting nonchemical, least-hazardous management alternatives.

Environmental Working Group | ewg.org

Analyzing government data, legal documents, and scientific studies, as well as conducting their own research to expose threats to public health and the environment and to find solutions.

Pesticide Action Network of North America | panna.org

Working to replace pesticide use with ecologically sound and socially just alternatives. The network promotes our right to know about chemicals used in our environment with consumer-friendly information on a range of toxics.

Public Citizen | citizen.org

Representing consumer interests in Congress, the executive branch, and the courts.

State PIRGS | pirg.org

Advocating for the public interest with an alliance of state-based, citizen-funded organizations.

Taking Precaution | takingprecaution.org

Providing an online hub for information about the precautionary principle.

Research and Education on Sustainable Agriculture and Genetically Modified Foods

Ag-Biotech Infonet | biotech-info.net

Providing links to current research and debates on the impacts and implications of agricultural biotechnology.

Institute for Responsible Technology | responsibletechnology.org

Offering educational resources about genetically modified foods, including books, newsletters, videos, and DVDs.

The Land Institute | landinstitute.org

Developing an agricultural system in balance with the ecological stability of the prairie and a grain yield comparable to that from annual crops.

Organic Center for Education and Promotion | organic-center.org

Providing scientific information about the benefits of organic food to consumers, health care professionals, educators, public officials, and government agencies.

Rodale Institute | rodaleinstitute.org

Promoting organic farming and conducting research on sustainable farming techniques. See newfarm.org for more resources from Rodale.

World Watch Institute | worldwatch.org

Conducting independent research for an environmentally sustainable and socially just society.

Resources for Chapter 2: Promoting Healthful Diets and Food Safety

Center for Food Safety | centerforfoodsafety.org

Challenging harmful food production technologies and promoting sustainable alternatives.

Center for Informed Food Choices | informedeating.org

Advocating for a diet based on whole, unprocessed, local, organically grown plant foods.

Center for Science in the Public Interest | cspinet.org

Advocating for nutrition and health, food safety, alcohol policy, and sound science. Check out their *Nutrition Action Health Letter* for resources on diet and health and tips on deciphering health claims in supermarkets, fast-food chains, and restaurants.

Consumers Union | consumersunion.org

Providing a comprehensive source for advice about products and services, personal finance, health and nutrition, and other consumer concerns. Check out GreenerChoices.org for tips on environmental consumption and Eco-Labels.org for information about many consumer labeling efforts.

Health Care without Harm | noharm.org

Bringing healthy food and other health-supporting practices into the medical industry.

Union of Concerned Scientists | ucsusa.org

A partnership of scientists and citizens combining scientific analysis, policy development, and citizen advocacy to achieve practical environmental solutions. Their Food and Environment Program promotes sustainable farming practices and is dedicated to phasing out the routine, nontherapeutic use of antibiotics in livestock and poultry.

Resources for Chapter 3: Ordering the Wake-Up Call

The Internet gives us nearly limitless information, but it can be misleading, as neutral-seeming but industry-funded websites spread through cyberspace. A few keystrokes and a little search engine prodding, though, can quickly get you to the truth. Anytime you visit an informational website spend a few minutes figuring out who is supporting the site before you explore further. Project Evergreen (projectevergreen.com), for instance, looks like an environmentally friendly organization promoting "the economic and environmental value of healthy, well-maintained green spaces." But dig a little on the Internet and you'll find its funding comes from some of the biggest agrichemical companies, including Dow AgroSciences, Syngenta, and TruGreen Chem-Lawn. Here are some online resources for doing web sleuthing of your own:

- **archives.org:** This site's "Wayback Machine" catalogues websites, going back to 1996. If you're looking into a company or organization that no longer has a website online or active, you might find it archived here.
- **ewg.org:** Online databases and research tools, including a resource section on agricultural subsidies and pesticide body burden.
- **guidestar.org:** Searchable financial and organizational data on all nonprofit organizations in the United States.
- **opensecrets.org:** Searchable database of political contributions and lobbying spending by individuals, corporations, and industries.
- **sourcewatch.org:** Background information on companies, front groups, and individuals.

Resources for Chapter 4: Promoting Grub

ORGANIC FOOD AND SUSTAINABLE FARMING

Center for Rural Affairs | cfra.org
Strengthening small businesses, family farms and ranches, and rural communities.

Community Alliance with Family Farmers | caff.org
Building a movement of rural and urban people to foster family-scale agriculture that cares for the land, sustains local economies, and promotes social justice.

Cornucopia Institute | cornucopia.org
Providing information to empower organic consumers in making good, discerning purchasing decisions, and serving as a government and corporate watchdog protecting the integrity of organic food.

Ecological Farming Association | eco-farm.org
Bringing together growers, activists, and industry-related businesses to exchange the latest advances in sustainable food production and marketing.

Family Farm Defenders | familyfarmdefenders.org
Working toward a farmer-controlled and consumer-oriented food system, based upon democratically controlled institutions that empower farmers to speak for and respect themselves.

Global Resource Action Center for the Environment | gracelinks.org
- **Factory Farm Project:** Ending factory farming as a means of production.
- **Sustainable Table:** Helping consumers make healthy food choices to create a sustainable system.
- **Eat Well Guide:** Providing information for local sources of sustainably raised meat, poultry, eggs, and dairy.

International Federation of Agriculture Movements | ifoam.org

Uniting and assisting the worldwide organic movement. A great resource for finding out how other countries are promoting organic production.

National Family Farm Coalition | nffc.net

Providing a voice for grassroots groups on farm, food, trade, and rural economic issues to ensure fair prices for family farmers, safe and healthy food, and vibrant, environmentally sound rural communities here and around the world.

Organic Consumers Association | organicconsumers.org

Building a national network of consumers promoting food safety, organic agriculture, fair trade, and sustainability. Their website includes ways to get involved with various campaigns in your community and around the country.

The True Food Network | truefoodnow.org

Linking citizens with campaigns and information on genetically engineered organisms through regular action alerts, updates, and access to their online resources.

LOCAL FOOD SYSTEMS: COMMUNITY-BASED EFFORTS

Center for Food and Justice | departments.oxy.edu/uepi/cfj/

Engaging in collaborative action, community capacity–building, and research and education to promote food justice. (A division of the Urban and Environmental Policy Institute at Occidental College.)

Community Food Security Coalition | foodsecurity.org

Building a strong, sustainable, local, and regional food system that ensures access to affordable, nutritious, and culturally appropriate food for all. Join their listserv, access their reports, and find other resources to engage with or start food security projects in your community.

FoodRoutes Network | foodroutes.org

Providing communications tools and information resources to help rebuild local, community-based food systems. Get resources to start a "Buy Fresh, Buy Local" campaign in your area.

Local Harvest | localharvest.org

Providing a comprehensive list of local food sources, CSAs, food coops, and more across the country. A really helpful resource for your Community Food Audit.

The Robyn Van En CSA Center | csacenter.org

Offering resources for starting CSAs or for supporting already existing CSAs.

LOCAL FOOD SYSTEMS: YOUTH-FOCUSED PROJECTS

b-healthy (New York City) | b-healthy.org

Educating low-income youth and youth workers about healthy cooking, nutrition, and affordable alternatives to low-quality school lunches, commercially processed junk food, and fast food.

The Food Project (Boston) | thefoodproject.org

A launching pad for new ideas about youth and adults partnering to create social change through sustainable agriculture.

Just Food (New York City) | justfood.org

Fostering a just and sustainable food system in New York City by developing new marketing and food-growing opportunities—including CSAs and urban farming—that address the needs of regional family farms and New York City community gardeners and neighborhoods.

The People's Grocery (Oakland) | peoplesgrocery.org

Supporting the right to healthy and affordable food and building community self-reliance by increasing neighborhood access to locally produced fruits and vegetables and by promoting social enterprise, youth entrepreneurship, sustainable agriculture, and grassroots organizing.

FAIR TRADE

Equal Exchange | equalexchange.org

Offering fair-trade and organic coffee, tea, sugar, cocoa, and chocolate produced by twenty-eight democratically run farm cooperatives located in fourteen countries in Latin America, Africa, and Asia.

Global Exchange | globalexchange.org
Promoting environmental, political, and social justice with a range of projects, from annual Green Festivals to fair-trade campaigns, to global reality tours, and more.

TransFair USA | transfairusa.org
Certifying fair-trade products in the United States since 1999. Includes information about how to find fair-trade products near you.

Via Campesina | viacampesina.org
Creating an international movement that coordinates peasant organizations of small- and middle-scale producers, agricultural workers, rural women, and indigenous communities across the globe.

JUST FOOD
Farmworker unions and farmworker advocacy organizations:
- Coalition of the Immokalee Workers | ciw-online.org
- Farm Labor Organizing Committee | floc.com
- Pineros y Campesinos Unidos del Noroeste (PCUN) | pcun.org
- United Farm Workers of America (UFW) | ufw.org
- Farmworker Justice Fund | fwjustice.org

National Black Farmers Association | blackfarmers.org
Supporting advocacy for land retention and rural development for black farmers and small-scale farmers to reverse the land loss of socially and economically disadvantaged farmers while creating economic opportunities for small farmers.

Oxfam America | oxfamamerica.org
Promoting the "Make Trade Fair" campaign and other projects to protect the rights of workers around the world and end hunger. Oxfam's "Change Initiative" supports a network of student leaders at colleges and universities in the United States.

Rural Coalition | ruralco.org
Advocating for policies that support a more just and sustainable food system and building an alliance of regionally and culturally diverse minority and small farmers, rural communities, and organizations.

Resources for Chapter 7: Out of the Kitchen, Into the Fire

Farm-to-College | farmtocollege.org
Connecting colleges and universities around the country that are promoting farm-to-college on their campuses.

Genetically Modified–Free Schools | www.gmfreeschools.org
Offering educational and campaign materials, including downloadable videos, how-to and media kits, purchasing directory, and other online support for groups working, training, and mentoring for GM-free schools.

Pesticide-Free Communities | beyondpesticides.org
Contact Beyond Pesticides to find out about groups in your area working to reduce pesticide use, or to learn how to start your own. In the Northeast, for instance, visit toxicsaction.org; in the Northwest, visit pesticide.org.

Pesticide-Free Schools | greenschools.net/index.html
Visit the Little Green Schoolhouse, which includes sample school board resolutions to get rid of toxics in your school.

Your Media Diet
A healthy diet is made up of not only the food you eat, but also the media you consume. Here are recommended books and magazines for trustworthy news and information about food, farming, and health as well as sources of inspirational stories about real change. Also, consider joining listservs from organizations you trust to get up-to-date news on the issues you care about.

- *Center for Media and Democracy SpinWatch* | prwatch.org
- *Nutrition Action Healthletter* from Center for Science in the Public Interest | cspinet.org
- *Orion Magazine* | oriononline.org
- *The Berkeley Wellness Letter* | berkeleywellness.com
- *WorldWatch Magazine* | worldwatch.org

BOOKS

We know the feeling: you arrive at a book's bibliography with every intention of pursuing further reading, but you're hit with an intimidating long list. While you may have had a genuine interest in delving deeper, your desire is quickly squashed by dear-old overwhelm. To give you a leg up, here is a selection of the top hits on Grub themes.

The Big Picture: Food Politics

Diet for a Dead Planet: How the Food Industry Is Killing Us, Christopher D. Cook

The corporation is a psychopath, so concludes the documentary *The Corporation* after administering the World Health Organization's personality diagnostic test. If so, the food industry is a particularly deadly one, with many in the United States dying or becoming sick from our diet. Investigative journalist Christopher Cook seeks to explain this phenomenon. Read this book and you will get the whole kit-and-caboodle analysis to help you make sense of our predicament.

Fast Food Nation: The Dark Side of the All-American Meal, Eric Schlosser

If you haven't already, join the three million-plus people who've read Schlosser's hard-hitting exposé. No longer is "non-fiction page-turner" an oxymoron. Schlosser introduces you to amazing characters—from the founders of the Golden Arches to the teenagers and minimum-wage workers who form the workforce for these corporate behemoths. You will never look at KFC, Wendy's, or McDonald's the same. And we think that's a very good thing.

Food Fight: The Inside Story of the Food Industry, America's Obesity Crisis, and What We Can Do About It, Kelly Brownell and Katherine Battle Horgen

Chock-full of statistics and zingers, this book is a great one-stop shop for understanding what is so unhealthy about the way we eat now, and what people are doing to try to change it.

Safe Food and *Food Politics*, Marion Nestle

New York University's Professor Marion Nestle is the country's best resource for understanding the nexus between food policy and the politics of food, and how the food industry has affected everything from the meat we eat to our national dietary guidelines. When her first book, *Food Politics*, hit the shelves, Nestle was slammed with a threatening letter from the U.S. Sugar Association (you can read it at: foodpolitics.com). You know you're touching a nerve when "big sugar" comes after you.

Trust Us, We're Experts! and *Toxic Sludge Is Good for You*,
John Stauber and Sheldon Rampton

Did you know that toxic sludge is actually good for you? Well, at least, that's what the Director of Public Information for the Water Environment Federation (formerly the Water Pollution Control Federation) wants you to think. "We're launching a campaign to get people to stop calling it sludge. We call it biosolids," she told John Stauber and Sheldon Rampton, co-authors of these alarming and eye-opening books about the public relations industry and its influence on public information. In a nation in which working public relations professionals now outnumber journalists, these books are required reading for the discerning citizen.

Diet, Health, and Our Food System

Eat, Drink, and Be Healthy: The Harvard Medical School Guide to Healthy Eating, Walter Willett, M.D., codeveloped with the Harvard School of Public Health

In a compelling, easy-to-follow manner, *Eat, Drink, and Be Healthy* explains the basic components of a healthy diet, including thorough information about fats, protein, carbohydrates, and why you should eat lots of fruits and vegetables. It also dispels dietary myths, including the over-hype about the need for dairy. Don't miss the great recipes buried in the back, which help put the book's lessons into culinary practice.

Our Stolen Future: Are We Threatening Our Fertility, Intelligence, and Survival? A Scientific Detective Story, Theo Colborn, Dianne Dumanoski, and John Peterson Myers

As important as Rachel Carson's *Silent Spring*, *Our Stolen Future* makes a powerful argument for the dangers of a new class of chemicals, endocrine disrupters. *Our Stolen Future* connects the dots between the hormone disruption of humans and animals and our toxic environment. It is also a call-to-arms for a profound overhaul of our regulatory systems and a precautionary approach to policymaking.

Seeds of Deception: Exposing Industry and Government Lies about the Safety of Genetically Engineered Foods, Jeffrey Smith

Be forewarned: after reading this book you may never want to eat processed foods containing GMOs again. Smith offers compelling detail about the science behind GMOs, the concerns scientists have raised about their health impact, and how these cautions have been silenced by industry.

Solutions

Eat Here: Reclaiming Homegrown Pleasures in a Global Supermarket, Brian Halweil

Brian Halweil offers up all the reasons to eat local, and examples of how people are doing it around the world. Halweil got his chops at the WorldWatch Institute, and this book is a culmination of work he did there. You'll turn the last page more inspired than ever to eat Grub.

Hope's Edge: The Next Diet for a Small Planet, Frances Moore Lappé and Anna Lappé

From the foothills of the Himalayas to villages in Bangladesh, from the central plains of Brazil to the rolling hills of western France, we explore the frontiers of citizen activism changing the face of food, farming, and economics. From a city in Brazil that declared access to good, healthy food a basic right of citizenship, to a grassroots network of farmers in India reclaiming their rights to seeds and organic farming, these vibrant, courageous movements have the collective power to change the course of history.

Raising Healthy Children in a Toxic World: 101 Smart Solutions for Every Family, Philip Landrigan, Herbert Needleman, Mary Landrigan

This handbook is a great source for tips about creating a healthy home and environment for you and your family. The book is a reminder that toxic exposure comes in many forms, not just in the food we ingest but also in the air we breathe, the water we drink, the playgrounds we hang out in, and the products we scour our bathtub with. And it's a toolkit for making those places—and more—the safest possible.

Contributors

CHEFS

Elizabeth Johnson is a food coach and wellness advisor to youth and adults in New York City where she works for b-healthy and Just Food. **b-healthy.org and justfood.org**

Ludie Minaya's travels led her to a love and respect for preserving food traditions. She shares her knowledge and passion with youth and adults as a program coordinator of b-healthy. **b-healthy.org**

Lara Comstock Oramas is a vegan whole foods chef interested in getting people to talk about and eat good, healthful food full of love and life. **leftoverscatering.com**

WINE SUGGESTIONS

Katrine Pollari is the owner of Olivino Wines in Brooklyn, New York. **olivinowines.com**

ARTISTS AND POETS

Suheir Hammad's latest collection of poems is *ZaatarDiva*, published fall 2005 by Cipher Books. **suheirhammad.com**

Tenjin Ikeda is an Afro–Puerto Rican artist born and raised in Brooklyn. He has been working in the art world for over seventeen years, in painting, sculpturing, and printmaking. **adesoji.com**

Dr. Marc Lappé was a nationally recognized expert on toxicology, medical ethics, genetics, and immunology. He was the founder of the Center for Ethics and Toxics in Gualala, California, where he helped start a community charter school. **cetos.org**

Michael Molina is an author and performance artist from New Orleans who works with young people in San Francisco to explore creative writing as a tool for personal healing and empowerment. **bluesborn.blogspot.com**

Matthew Willse is a Brooklyn-based designer who prefers collaborators over clients and believes that small revolutions are the way to go. **thecoup.org**

SOUNDTRACKS

Laurent "Tippy" Alfred is a musician, activist, teacher, and father from St. Croix who, along with his queen Selam, owns and operates I Grade Records, a reggae music label committed to producing and releasing the highest quality roots music from the Virgin Islands. **igraderecords.com**

Peter Berley is the author of *Fresh Food Fast* and *The Modern Vegetarian Kitchen*. **peterberley.com**

Annemarie Colbin is an author and health educator and the founder of the Natural Gourmet Cookery School/Institute for Food and Health. **foodandhealing.com**

DJ Reborn is deeply committed to music, knowledge, food, and laughter.

Lila Downs was born in the mountains of Oaxaca the daughter of a Mixtec Indian woman and Anglo-American father. She unites cultures and boundaries with her extraordinary voice. **liladowns.com**

Bobbito Garcia is the editor-in-chief of *Bounce: From the Playground*, a *Vibe* magazine music columnist, and the author of *Where'd You Get Those? NYC's Sneaker Culture 1960–1987*. He is also a DJ and basketball performer. **somosarte.com/bobbito**

Jessica B. Harris is a food historian and the author of nine cookbooks detailing the foods of the African diaspora. **africooks.com**

Robin D. G. Kelly is the author of several books, most recently *Freedom Dreams: The Black Radical Imagination.* He is completing a biography of Thelonious Monk.

Bruce Mack is a music educator and member of the expressionist bands Burnt Sugar and Tricky Dilemma. His work as a performer and activist for the advancement of black musicians creating music outside the box has been documented in the book *The Right to Rock: The Black Rock Coalition and the Cultural Politics of Race.* **brucemack.com**

Evon Peter is Neetsaii Gwich'in from Artic Village in northeastern Alaska. He has just fulfilled three years as the chief for his tribe. He is cochair to the Gwich'in Council International, chairman of Native Movement, and on the executive board of the Alaska Inter-tribal Council. **nativemovement.org**

James Spooner is the director of the film *Afro-Punk.* **afropunk.com**

Research

Judith Belasco believes that food transforms the world. She is a master's degree candidate in nutrition at Teachers College, Columbia University. She writes about food and nutrition from her home in Brooklyn, New York.

Erin Caricofe explores cuisine through its many lenses: formal culinary training, cultural studies, nutrition and health trends, children's education, and, of course, sensory delight. In interviewing farmers for *Grub,* she met fascinating, passionate souls, and found herself feeling closer to her country than ever before.

Sara Safransky is cofounder of Maverick Farms, a sustainable-agriculture nonprofit and working farm in the Blue Ridge Mountains of western North Carolina, where she and her fellow farmers are helping reclaim the pleasures of eating and sharing meals in a culture overrun by flavorless food. They love visitors. **maverickfarms.org**

Acknowledgments

We are grateful to our agents, Jim Levine and Arielle Eckstut, at Levine Greenberg, edifying from day one. At Tarcher/Penguin, we are thankful to our wonderful team, including publisher Joel Fotinos and executive editor Mitch Horowitz, who believed in the project from its inception and offered his sage advice, over and above the call of duty. Additional thanks are due to associate editor Ashley Shelby for her consistent support and uncanny eye for detail.

Special thanks to our first Grub party hosts and our party guinea pigs. They were all great sports.

And a shout out to Tillie's, where it all got started.

BRYANT TERRY AND ANNA LAPPÉ

FROM BRYANT

I give thanks to the following:

To the Creator, my angels, and my ancestors (upon your shoulders I stand) for your guidance.

To my grandparents, especially the late Margie Bryant (Ma'Dear) and the late Andrew Johnson Terry I (Paw Paw) for your love of food that you passed on to me.

To my parents, Beatrice and Booker Terry, and my sister, Jamelah Terry, for your unwavering belief in and support of me (no matter how eccentric I am). You're my foundation.

To all my extended family members—the Bryants and the Terrys.

To Bethanie Hines for your love, consistent support, inspiration, and feedback on my food. You are a gift from the creator who constantly reminds me to give thanks, be present, cocreate my life, and love hard.

To Gale, Foster, and Amber Hines for your enthusiastic support and love.

To Ludie Minaya, Elizabeth Johnson, and Latham Thomas for caring about b-healthy as much as I do and for being beautiful friends.

To all the past, present, and future b-healthy youth. You are the future of this food justice movement.

To Lara Comstock for your friendship and the invaluable experience I gained catering with you.

To Leda Scheintaub for being an *amazing* recipe tester, copy editor, and friend.

To all my teachers and mentors for your wisdom and guidance. Special thanks to Annemarie Colbin for your encouragement and Peter Berley for your advice early on.

To all those who supported me at Xavier University of Louisiana, New York University, and the Natural Gourmet Cookery School.

To my talented friends who contributed soundtracks and artwork to complement my menus.

To my New York crew (Beacon included)—some of the most remarkable artists, activists, educators, and healers on the planet—you constantly inspire me. Big-up to Planet Brooklyn! To my Bay Area crew (Santa Cruz included)—you constantly remind me of what's really important (fresh air, water, trees, mountains, and slowing down). Peace to my new home Oaktown.

For the historical record, Anna Lappé is one of the smartest, coolest, and most creative people on this planet. Thanks for being a friend, mentor, and cocreator. And thanks for finding me . . .

FROM ANNA

My deep appreciation to the dozens and dozens of farmers and scientists, food activists and researchers, and public health advocates and policymakers interviewed for this book who are at the front lines of making Grub-for-all a reality. I am grateful for your assistance, awed by your work, and moved by your commitment. I am especially indebted to the farmers, particularly DeLisa Lewis, who gave me an insider's view of life on an organic farm.

My gratitude, also, to insight and inspiration from colleagues at the Food and Society Policy Fellows Program of the WK Kellogg Foundation.

The following organizations provided essential research: the Center for Media and Democracy, Community Food Security Coalition, Consumers Union (especially Urvashi Rangan, PhD), Environmental Working Group, Institute for Agriculture and Trade Policy, Natural Resources Defense Council, Organic Consumers Association, Organic Farming and Research Foundation, and Pesticide Action Network of North America. (Of course, the views—and any errors—in this book are mine alone.)

Additional thanks to advice and inspiration from those bringing Grub to life in their restaurants and businesses, particularly Dan Barber of Blue Hill, Mary Cleaver of Cleaver Co., Didi Emmons of Veggie Planet, Leslie MacEarhern of Angelica Kitchen, Patrick Martins and Todd Wickstrom of Heritage Foods USA, and Bart Potenza and Joy Pierson of Candle Café.

Eric Schlosser offered his support back when this book was only a title. Thank you.

My thanks also to Judith Belasco and Sara Safransky for your stellar research assistance, to Erin Caricofe for your invaluable interviews with organic farmers throughout the country, to Matthew Willse for your brilliant graphics, and to Zoe Rosenfeld and Hope Richardson for your essential editorial support. My appreciation to Richard Rowe for priceless feedback. And to Paul Mailman for a patient and loving ear. I am forever indebted.

Special thanks to Sadie Kaufman and Rena Mundo. You helped me tap the joy in this work, and saved me in the process. This book is unquestionably better because of you. And to my friends across the country who, once again, let me crash on their actual (and proverbial) couches, especially Danny Anisfeld, Ellen Berrey, Jessica Walker Beaumont and Sidney Beaumont, Gita Drury, Kate Hallward, and Rebekah Rutkoff.

To my brothers and sisters and to Jacki Lappé, your support has meant everything to me.

A toast to Bryant Terry, who has become family: here's to many more delectable meals, stimulating conversations, and big dreams.

This book would not have been possible without the consistent love—not to mention eagle-eyed editing—of my mother, Frances Moore Lappé, who has always, and unflaggingly, believed in me. What a journey, Mom.

I dedicate this book to my father, Marc Alan Lappé, a lifelong question-asker, storyteller, and teacher. His life embodied an unswerving commitment to standing up to powerful corporate interests with concern for those most vulnerable to toxics in our environment. He did so with unfaltering integrity and a poet's heart. The planet misses you. I miss you.

Notes

CHAPTER 1: THE SIX ILLUSIONS

1. Barbara Kingsolver, "A Good Farmer," *The Nation,* excerpt from *The Essential Agrarian Reader,* November 3, 2003, 11–18.

2. Mark Nord, Margaret Andrews, and Steven Carlson, "Household Food Security in the United States, 2003," *Food Assistance and Nutrition Research Report* No. 42, U.S. Department of Agriculture (USDA), Economic Research Service (ERS), October 2004, 6.

3. From USDA Economic Research Service. Total food availability in the United States is estimated at 3,900 calories per person per day. See, for example, David M. Cutler, Edward L. Glaeser, and Jesse M. Shapiro, "Why Have Americans Become More Obese?" *The Economics of Obesity* / E-FAN-04-004, USDA ERS, April 2004.

4. In 1970, there were 2,780,000 farms; in 2002, 1,909,598. From USDA ERS.

5. Thomas A. Lyson, *Civic Agriculture: Reconnecting Farm, Food, and Community* (Lebanon, NH: Tufts University Press, 2004), 42.

6. The National Institute for Occupational Safety and Health (NIOSH) reports the suicide rate for farmers is double the national average rate. See, for instance, "Farmer Suicides: A Ten Year Analysis in Three Southeastern States." Available at www.cdc.gov/niosh.

7. According to the National Farm Medicine Center (Marshfield, Wisconsin), www.marshfieldclinic.org.

8. Latest figures from the EPA: "Pesticide Sales and Usage: 2000 and 2001 Market Estimates," Office of Pesticide Programs, May 2004. Available at www.epa.gov/oppbead1/pestsales/.

9. Author communication, Dr. David Pimentel, August 2004. See, for instance, David Pimentel et al., "Environmental and Economic Impacts of Reducing U.S. Agricultural Pesticide Use" in David Pimentel and A.A. Hanson, eds., *CRC Handbook of Pest Management in Agriculture,* 2nd edition, Volume 1 (Boca Raton, FL: CRC Press, Inc., 1991).

10. In 2005, controversy flared over the number of deaths attributable to obesity-related illnesses. The Centers for Disease Control estimated that 365,000 people die every year from obesity-related illnesses (*Journal of the American Medical Association* 2005; 293: 298), but in April 2005, researchers using a different methodology lowered the estimate to 111,909 (Katherine Flegal et al., "Excess Deaths Associated with Underweight, Overweight, and Obesity," *Journal of the American Medical Association,* April 20, 2005, 293(15): 1918–9). Despite the Flegal findings, Dr. Walter Willett at the Harvard School of Public Health, one of the nation's leading experts on obesity, diet, and health, contends that 365,000 deaths per year due to obesity-related illnesses is still an accurate estimate. (Obesity is determined by your body mass index [BMI], a measurement of your height and weight. A woman my height, 5'6", for instance, would be obese if she weighed 186 pounds or more. BMI index available at: www.cdc.gov/nccdphp/dnpa/bmi/calc-bmi.htm.)

11. See Note 10.

12. Andrew Kimbrell, ed., *Fatal Harvest: The Tragedy of Industrial Agriculture* (Washington, D.C.: Island Press, 2002), 79.

13. Ibid., 75, 77.

14. See, for instance, Felipe Fernandez-Armesto, *Food: A History* (London, England: Pan Macmillan, 2002).

15. Figures on percentage GMO crops latest as of June 2005. See Jeffrey Smith, *Seeds of Deception: Exposing Industry and Government Lies about the Safety of Genetically Engineered Foods* (Fairfield, IA: Yes! Books, 2003).

16. Survey opinion from William K. Hallman, PhD, et al. "Public Perceptions of Genetically Modified Foods: A National Study of American Knowledge and Opinion," Food Policy Institute, Rutgers–The State University of New Jersey, October 2003, Executive Summary, 1. Data on countries planting GMOs from the International Service for the Acquisition of Agri-biotech Applications, www.isaaa.org. China labeling required by Decree No. 10 of the Ministry of Agriculture in January 2002, from the Center for Food Safety, "Genetically Engineered Crops and Foods: Worldwide Regulation and Prohibition," July 2005. Available at www.center forfoodsafety.org.

17. From CropLife America Annual Meeting Registrants, as of September 8, 2004.

18. John Wargo, *Our Children's Toxic Legacy: How Science and Law Fail to Protect Us from Pesticides* (New Haven, CT: Yale University Press, Second Edition, 1998), 29. Malaria killed more troops than those who died in combat. In the 1930s alone, 50 million people died from malaria.

19. Theo Colborn, John Peterson Myers, and Dianne Dumanoski, *Our Stolen Future* (New York: Plume Books, 1997), 200.

20. Ibid., 200.

21. From the National Agricultural Aviation Association. Accessible at: www.agaviation.org.

22. Latest figures from the EPA: "Pesticide Sales and Usage: 2000 and 2001 Market Estimates," Office of Pesticide Programs, May 2004. Available at www.epa.gov/oppbead1/pestsales/.

23. The Centers for Disease Control and Prevention, "The Third National Report on Human Exposure to Environmental Chemicals," July 2005. Available at www.cdc.gov/exposurereport. See an analysis of the CDC study in "Chemical Trespass: Pesticides in Our Bodies and Corporate Accountability" (San Francisco, CA: Pesticide Action Network of North America, 2004). Available at www.panna.org.

24. Environmental Working Group, "Body Burden: The Pollution in Newborns" (Washington, D.C.: EWG), July 14, 2005. Available at www.ewg.org. See also, Colborn, Myers, and Dumanoski, *Our Stolen Future,* 240.

25. Author communication with Senior Investigator of the Agricultural Health Study, Dr. Michael C.R. Alavanja, January 2005. For instance, Agricultural Health Study researchers have found that farmers using methyl bromide had a 41 percent increased risk of prostate cancer. See also, Dan Fagin, Marianne Lavelle, and the Center for Public Integrity, *Toxic Deception: How the Chemical Industry Manipulates Science, Bends the Law, and Endangers Your Health* (Monroe, ME: Common Courage Press, 1999), xvi.

26. See for instance, Ted Schettler, Gina Solomon, Maria Valenti, Annette Huddle, *Generations at Risk: Reproductive Health and the Environment* (Cambridge, MA: MIT Press, 2000), 117–18. See also, "Pesticides: Improvements Needed to Ensure the Safety of Farmworkers and Their Children," Government Accountability Office, Report to Congressional Requesters, GAO/RCED-00-40, March 2000, especially pages 5 and 14.

27. See for instance, United Nations Food and Agriculture Organization, "Children Face Higher Risks from Pesticide Poisoning," October 5, 2001. Available at www.fao.org. See also, Wargo, *Our Children's Toxic Legacy,* 178.

28. See, for instance, the findings of the Geoparkinson Study, Anthony Seaton of the University of Aberdeen, UK, principal investigator, funded by the European Commission. Available at www.abdn.ac.uk/deom/geop.shtml. See also Andy Coghlan, "Exposure to Pesticides Can Cause Parkinson's," *New Scientist,* Issue 2501, May 26, 2005, 14.

29. See for instance, Shanna Swan, Ph.D., and the Study for the Future of Families Research Group et al., "Semen Quality in Relation to Biomarkers of Pesticide Exposure," *Environmental Health Perspectives,* Vol. 11, No. 12, September 2003, 1478–1484. See also, Shanna Swan, Ph.D., et al., "Geographic Differences in Semen Quality of Fertile U.S. Males," *Environmental Health Perspectives,* Vol. 11, No. 4, April 2003, 414–420. Other studies can be found at www.ourstolenfuture.org.

30. Rates of childhood cancer from Schettler et al., *Generations at Risk,* 120. See also S. H. Zahm and M. H. Ward, "Pesticides and Childhood Cancer," *Environmental Health Perspectives,* June 1998; 106 Suppl 3:893–908. See also, "Pesticides: Improvements Needed to Ensure the Safety of Farmworkers and Their Children," Government Accountability Office, Report to Congressional Requesters, GAO/RCED-00-40, March 2000, 5.

31. Wargo, *Our Children's Toxic Legacy,* 3.

32. Ibid., 75.

33. Latest figures from the EPA: "Pesticide Sales and Usage: 2000 and 2001 Market Estimates," Office of Pesticide Programs, May 2004. Available at www.epa.gov/oppbead1/pestsales/.

34. For a comprehensive study of the impact of pesticides, read John Wargo, *Our Children's Toxic Legacy.*

35. Wargo, *Our Children's Toxic Legacy,* 57. See also National Academy of Sciences, "The Future Role of Pesticides in U.S. Agriculture," Commission on Life Sciences (Washington, D.C.: National Academy Press, 2000), 25.

36. Colborn et al., *Our Stolen Future,* 197.

37. Rachel Carson, *Silent Spring* (Boston: Houghton Mifflin, 1962), 6. Quoted in Gina Solomon and A. M. Huddle, "Low Levels of Persistent Organic Pollutants Raise Concerns for Future Generations," *Journal of Epidemiological Community Health,* 2002; 56: 826–827.

38. From EPA. Available at www.epa.gov/pesticides/food/risks.htm.

39. Colborn et al., *Our Stolen Future,* 217.

40. Crops using benomyl: According to "Benomyl Cancellation Request Published," EPA, June 13, 2001. Available at www.epa.gov/oppfead1/cb/csb_page/updates/benomylcl.htm. Health effects of benomyl: Wargo, *Our Children's Toxic Legacy,* 11, 221.

41. Antony Barnett, "Eyeless Children Championed by Observer Win $7m Test Case," *The Observer,* December 21, 2003. Available at www.observer.co.uk.

42. Wargo, *Our Children's Toxic Legacy,* 220.

43. Ibid., 222.

44. Barnett, "Eyeless Children."

45. Ibid.

46. Ibid.

47. "Benomyl Cancellation Request Published," EPA, June 13, 2001. Jim Borel, a DuPont vice president and general manager for DuPont Crop Protection, stating: "A significant element of the reason to withdraw is that the company is no longer willing to bear the high and continuing costs of defending the product in the U.S. legal system where factors other than good science can influence outcomes." Quoted in "DuPont Phases Out Benlate Sales," Civil RICO Report, Vol. 17, No. 1, May 9, 2001.

48. "Benomyl Cancellation Order Published," EPA, August 10, 2001. Available at www.epa.gov/oppfead1/cb/csb_page/updates/benomylcanc.htm.

49. Federal Insecticide, Fungicide, and Rodenticide Act U.S.C. §§ 136–136y, June 25, 1947, as amended 1972, 1973, 1975, 1978, 1983, 1984, 1988, 1990, 1991, and 1996. Viewable at http://ipl.unm.edu/cwl/fedbook/fifra.html.

50. Wargo, *Our Children's Toxic Legacy,* xii.

51. Paracelsus quoted by Rutgers University Professor Joe Rosen at an American Chemistry Society meeting, Summer 2004.

52. Schettler et al., *Generations at Risk,* 108.

53. Based on the latest lists from the EPA, "Inert (other) Pesticide Ingredients in Pesticide Products." Viewable at www.epa.gov/opprd001/inerts/lists.html. Toxicity of List 4b inerts from author communication with Natural Resources Defense Council and Northwest Coalition for Alternatives to Pesticides, July 2005.

54. National Academy of Sciences, *Pesticides in the Diets of Infants and Children* (Washington, D.C.: National Academy Press, 1993) 4.

55. Frederick S. vom Saal and Claude Hughes, "An Extensive New Literature Concerning Low-Dose Effects of Bisphenol A Shows the Need for a New Risk Assessment," *Environmental Health Perspectives,* August 2005, Vol. 113, No. 8, 926–933.

56. On List 3 as of July 2005: www.epa.gov/opprd001/inerts.

57. "Pesticides: Improvements Needed to Ensure the Safety of Farmworkers and Their Children," Government Accountability Office, GAO/RCED-00-40, March 2000, 4.

58. Ibid., 4.

59. See, for instance, Colborn et al., *Our Stolen Future,* 229.

60. Syngenta reports terbuthylazine use in Europe on its website, www.syngentacropprotection-us.com.

61. See, for instance, Jules Pretty and Rachel Hine, "Reducing Food Poverty with Sustainable Agriculture," Center for Environment and Society, University of Essex, UK, February, 2001. Available at www2.essex.ac.uk/ces/Research Programmes/SAFEWexecsummfinalreport.htm.

62. From the documentary *Meat* (dir. Frederick Wiseman, 1979).

63. Quoted in Wargo, *Our Children's Toxic Legacy,* 81.

64. Ibid., 14.

65. Quoted in the preface of Robert van den Bosch, *The Pesticide Conspiracy* (Berkeley, CA: University of California Press, 1989), xv.

66. David Pimentel et al., "Environmental and Economic Impacts of Reducing U.S. Agricultural Pesticide Use," in David Pimentel and A. A. Hanson, eds., *CRC Handbook of Pest Management in Agriculture,* 2nd edition, Volume 1 (Boca Raton, FL: CRC Press, Inc., 1991).

67. Wargo, *Our Children's Toxic Legacy,* 7. Quoting Dr. David Pimentel.

68. Author communication, Dr. David Pimentel, August 2004.

69. Donald. W. Lotter, "Organic Agriculture," *Journal of Sustainable Agriculture,* Vol. 21, Issue 4, 2003, 19. Available at www.donlotter.net.

70. Erica Walz, "Final Results of the Fourth National Organic Farmers' Survey: Sustaining Organic Farms in a Changing Organic Marketplace," Organic Farming and Research Foundation, 2004, 20. Available online at www.ofrf.org.

71. USDA Agricultural Research Service, Methyl Bromide Factsheet.

72. See Frances Moore Lappé, *Diet for a Small Planet* (20th Anniversary Edition) (New York: Ballantine Books, 1991).

73. See, for instance, David Pimentel, Laura Westra, and Reed Noss, eds., *Ecological Integrity: Integrating Environment, Conservation and Health* (Washington, D.C.: Island Press, 2001).

74. Timothy W. Jones, Ph.D., "Using Contemporary Archaeology and Applied Anthropology to Understand Food Loss in the American Food System," Bureau of Applied Research in Anthropology, University of Arizona, 2004.

75. Erin M. Tegtmeier and Michael D. Duffy, Department of Economics, Iowa State University, Ames, Iowa, "External Costs of Agricultural Production in the United States," *International Journal of Agricultural Sustainability*, Vol. 2, No. 1, 2004. See also, the USGS, "Contamination of Water in the Midcontinental United States from Pesticide Application to Row Crops (Corn and Soybeans) Has Been a Major Water-Quality Issue During the Past Decade." Available at ks.water.usgs.gov.

76. From Environmental Defense. Available at www.scorecard.org.

77. Ibid.

78. Tegtmeier et al., "External Costs," 16.

79. See Farm Subsidy Database from the Environmental Working Group. Available at www.ewg.org.

80. Christopher D. Cook, *Diet for a Dead Planet: How the Food Industry Is Killing Us* (New York: The New Press, 2004), 5. Quoting Dr. David Pimentel and Dr. Mario Giampietro, "Food, Land, Population and the U.S. Economy," November 21, 1994.

81. Richard Manning, "The Oil We Eat: Following the Food Chain Back to Iraq," *Harper's Magazine,* February 2004. Available at http://harpers.org/TheOilWeEat.html.

82. "Deception in Weight-Loss Advertising Workshop: Seizing Opportunities and Building Partnerships to Stop Weight-Loss Fraud," Federal Trade Commission, Washington, D.C., December 2003, 32. Homeland security budget from "Historical Tables," Budget of the United States Government, Fiscal Year 2006, Office of Management and Budget, Washington, D.C., 2005, 80.

83. Andrew L. Dannenberg, Deron C. Burton, and Richard J. Jackson, "Economic and Environmental Costs of Obesity: The Impact on Airlines," National Center for Environmental Health, Centers for Disease Control and Prevention, Atlanta, Georgia, *American Journal of Preventive Medicine,* September 23, 2004, Vol. 27, No. 3, 264.

84. Eric A. Finkelstein, Ian Fiebelkorn, and Guijing Wang, "State-Level Estimates of Annual Medical Expenditures Attributable to Obesity," *Obesity Research,* North American Association for the Study of Obesity, January 2004, Vol. 12, No. 1: 18–24. In 2003, an estimated $75 billion was spent to treat obesity-related medical problems; half of this was financed by Medicaid or Medicare. Available at www.obesityresearch.org/cgi/reprint/12/1/18. See also, Kenneth E. Thorpe et al., "The Rising Prevalence of Treated Disease: Effects on Private Health Insurance Spending," *Health Affairs,* June 27, 2005, 317–325.

85. Presented at American Agricultural Economics Association Workshop, "Policy Issues in the Changing Structure of the Food System," July 29, 2000. Charles F. Curtiss, Iowa State University, Ames, Iowa. Neil E.

Harl, "The Age of Contract Agriculture," *Journal of Agribusiness,* Vol. 18, No. 1, March, 2000, 115–127. See also, Neil Harl, "Antitrust Issues in the New Food System," available at www.farmfoundation.org/tampa/harl.pdf.

86. Campbell R. McConnell and Stanley L. Brue, *Economics,* 16th edition (New York: McGraw-Hill/Irwin, 2005), 468.

87. Mary Hendrickson and William Heffernan, "Concentration of Agricultural Markets," Department of Rural Sociology, University of Missouri, January 2005. Available at www.foodcircles.missouri.edu.

88. Ibid.

89. Quoted on homepage for the Communiqué: "Oligopoly, Inc.: Concentration in Corporate Power," (Ottawa, Canada: Action Group on Erosion, Technology and Concentration, 2003). Accessed on April 5, 2005 at www.etcgroup.org/article.asp?newsid=420.

90. ActionAid International, "Power Hungry: Six Reasons to Regulate Global Food Corporations," (Johannesburg, South Africa: Action Aid), 13.

91. Ibid., 13.

92. Hendrickson and Heffernan, "Concentration of Agricultural Markets."

93. "Wal-Mart Food: Big, and Getting Bigger," *Retail Forward,* September 2003. Accessed on April 5, 2005 at www.retailforward.com/freecontent/Walmart_food.asp.

94. Kimberly Morland, Steve Wing, Ana Diez Roux, and Charles Poole, "Neighborhood Characteristics Associated with the Location of Food Stores and Food Service Places," *American Journal of Preventive Medicine,* January 2002, 22(1), 23–9.

95. Tracie McMillan, "The Action Diet: Get Better Food in Your Neighborhood," *City Limits,* July/August 2004. Available at www.citylimits.org. In New York City, the top 74,000 wealthiest New Yorkers have more than five square feet of grocery stores apiece; 1.6 million of the poorest have less than one.

96. Cook, *Diet for a Dead Planet,* 23.

97. Federal Trade Commission Staff Study, "Slotting Allowances in the Retail Grocery Industry: Selected Case Studies in Five Product Categories," November 2003. Available at www.ftc.gov.

98. Kurt Eichenwald, "Archer Daniels Settles Suit Accusing It of Price Fixing," *The New York Times,* June 18, 2004, C3.

99. Ibid.

100. The Associated Press, "Archer Daniels Midland to Pay $400 Million to Settle Corn Sweetener Lawsuit," June 17, 2004, BC cycle, state and local wire.

101. ActionAid International, *Power Hungry,* 5.

102. American Antitrust Institute, "Antitrust Fares Relatively Well in President's FY 2003 Budget, but Slowing Merger Pace Can Spell a Problem," February 13, 2002. Available at www.antitrustinstitute.org. Kevin J. Clancy and Peter C. Krieg, "Surviving Innovation: Common Testing Mistakes Can Derail a Promising New Product Launch," *Marketing Management,* March–April 2003. Available at www.copernicusmarketing.com.

103. James Bovard, "Archer Daniels Midland: A Case Study in Corporate Welfare," Policy Analysis, Cato Policy Analysis No. 241, September 26, 1995, 1. Accessed at www.cato.org/pubs/pas/pa-241.html.

104. In 2003, total farm subsidies were $16.4 billion. All data from Environmental Working Group, Farm Subsidy Database. Available at www.ewg.org/farm.

105. Environmental Working Group's Farm Subsidy Database.

106. Bovard, "Archer Daniels Midland."

107. Thomas A. Lyson, *Civic Agriculture: Reconnecting Farm, Food, and Community* (Lebanon, NH: Tufts University Press, 2004), 42.

108. Poultry statistics from Dr. C. Robert Taylor, Auburn University, an expert on contract farming. Vegetable contracts from Lyson, *Civic Agriculture,* 42.

109. Author communication, C. Robert Taylor, December 2004. See also, C. Robert Taylor, "Agricultural and Resource Policy Forum Restoring Economic Health to Contract Poultry Production," Taylor Auburn University College of Agriculture, May 2002.

110. Ibid. Quoting: *U.S. v. Trans-Missouri Freight Association,* 166 U.S. 290, 323–324 (1897).

111. William K. Hallman, Ph.D., W. Carl Hebden, Helen L. Aquino, Cara L. Cuite, Ph.D., and John T. Lang, "Public Perceptions of Genetically Modified Foods: A National Study of American Knowledge and Opinion," Food Policy Institute, Rutgers–The State University of New Jersey, October 2003, 1.

112. See for instance, Jeffrey Smith, *Genetic Roulette: The Documented Health Risks of Genetically Engineered Foods* (Fairfield, IA: Yes! Books, 2005). See also, Smith's *Seeds of Deception,* and Mae-Wan Ho, *GMO Free: Exposing the Hazards of Biotechnology to Ensure the Integrity of Our Food Supply* (Danbury, CT: Vital Health Publishing, 2004).

113. See Jessa Netting and Linda Wang, "The Newly Sequenced Genome Bares All," *Science News,* Vol. 159, No. 7, February 17, 2001, 100. See also, Barry Commoner, "Unraveling the DNA Myth: The Spurious Foundation of Genetic Engineering," *Harper's Magazine,* February 2002.

114. Commoner, "Unraveling the DNA Myth."

115. Ibid.

116. Author communication, Mark Lipson, Organic Research and Farming Association, June 2005.

117. "Genetically Modified Corn Concerns," *The Globe and Mail,* June 2, 2005, online edition, www.globeandmail.com.

118. Geoffrey Lean, "Revealed: Health Fears Over Secret Study Into GM Food; Rats Fed GM Corn Developed Abnormalities In Blood and Kidneys," *The Independent,* May 25, 2005, 6–7 and 26.

119. See, Michael S. Rosenwald, "Syngenta Says It Sold Wrong Biotech Corn," *Washington Post,* March 23, 2005, E01. See also, Paul Elias, "Tons of Experimental Biotech Corn Inadvertently Shipped to Farmers," *Associated Press,* March 23, 2005.

120. Jonathan Birchall, "Monsanto Agrees to U.S. $1.5m Penalty Over Crop Bribe," *Financial Times,* January 7, 2005, 4.

121. Center for Food Safety, "Monsanto vs. U.S. Farmers" (Washington, D.C.: Center for Food Safety, 2005), 4.

122. Ibid., 4.

123. Ibid., Executive Summary.

CHAPTER 2: THE (NOT SO) GREAT AMERICAN EXPERIMENT

1. A. Elizabeth Sloan, "Top 10 Global Food Trends," *FoodTechnology,* April 2005, Vol. 59, No. 4, 21.

2. Jane Goodall and Gary McAvoy, *Harvest for Hope: A Guide to Mindful Eating* (New York: Warner Books, forthcoming 2006), from unpublished manuscript.

3. Craig Lambert, "The Way We Eat Now: Ancient Bodies Collide with Modern Technology to Produce a Flabby, Disease-Ridden Populace," *Harvard Magazine,* May–June 2004: Vol. 106, No. 5, 50.

4. Judy Putnam, Jane Allshouse, and Linda Scott, "U.S. Per Capita Food Supply Trends: More Calories, Refined Carbohydrates, and Fats," *Food Review,* Winter 2002, Vol. 25, Issue 3, 2.

5. Ibid., 10. (Over the age of 2, from CSFII data from 1994–96.)

6. 5-A-Day Program, "Fruit and Vegetable Intake in the U.S. Survey Data and Demographics." Accessed March 15, 2005 at www.5aday.com/html/research/consumptionstats.php#highlights.

7. Ibid.

8. Feeding Infant and Toddler Study (FITS) quoted in Bonnie Sherman, "Teaching Baby to Eat," Colorado State University, May 11, 2004. Accessed at http://www.ext.colostate.edu/pubs/columncc/cc040511.html.

9. Putnam et al., "U.S. Per Capita Food Supply Trends," 10–11.

10. Ibid. See also, George Bray, Samara Joy Nielsen, and Barry M. Popkin, "Consumption of High-Fructose Corn Syrup in Beverages May Play a Role in the Epidemic of Obesity," *American Society for Clinical Nutrition,* 2004; 79:537–43.

11. 223 pounds figure from 2004, Economic Research Service, USDA, Agricultural Baseline Projections: U.S. Livestock, 2005–2014. Accessed April 10, 2005, at www.ers.usda.gov/Briefing/Baseline/livstk.htm. Figures on factory-farmed meat based on estimates of organic meat in the United States by the USDA ERS "Harmony Between Agriculture and the Environment: Current Issues," August 17, 2001. Accessed at www .ers.usda.gov/Emphases/Harmony/issues/organic/organic.html.

12. Putnam et al., "U.S. Per Capita Food Supply Trends."

13. Michael Jacobsen, Ph.D., "The Forgotten Killer . . . and FDA's Failure to Protect the Public's Health," (Washington, D.C.: Center for Science in the Public Interest), February 2005, iv.

14. See Note 11.

15. Red meat consumption down, from Putnam, et al., "U.S. Per Capita Food Supply Trends."

16. Consumer Policy and Consumer Health Protection Directorate, "Opinion of the Scientific Committee on Veterinary Measures Relating to Public Health Assessment of Potential Risks to Human Health from Hormone Residues in Bovine Meat and Meat Products," European Commission, April 30, 1999. These findings were reconfirmed in a 2002 report that reexamined the findings of seventeen studies reviewing this issue: European

Commission, Health and Consumer Protection Directorate-General, "Opinion of the Scientific Committee on Veterinary Measures Relating to Public Health on Review of Previous SCVPH Opinions of April 30, 1999 and May 3, 2000 on the Potential Risks to Human Health from Hormone Residues in Bovine Meat and Meat Products," European Commission, April 10, 2002.

17. Margaret Mellon, Charles Benbrook, and Karen Lutz Benbrook, "Hogging It: Estimates of Antimicrobial Abuse in Livestock" (Boston, MA: Union of Concerned Scientists, 2001). Accessed at www.ucsusa.org.

18. Ibid.

19. National Institute of Allergy and Infectious Diseases, National Institutes of Health, U.S. Department of Health and Human Services. Accessed at www.niaid.nih.gov/factsheets/antimicro.htm.

20. Amy Chapin, Ana Rule, Kristen Gibson, Timothy Buckley, and Kellogg Schwab, "Airborne Multidrug-Resistant Bacteria Isolated from a Concentrated Swine Feeding Operation," *Environmental Health Perspectives,* Vol. 13, No. 2, February 2005, Abstract.

21. Bray et al., "Consumption of High-Fructose Corn Syrup," 79: 537–43.

22. Greg Critser, *Fat Land: How Americans Became the Fattest People in the World* (Boston, MA: Mariner Books, 2004), 10.

23. Ibid., 18.

24. The FDA ruled on GRAS originally in 1983 and reaffirmed the ruling in 1996 in Reg. 43447: "Direct Food Substances Affirmed as Generally Recognized as Safe; High Fructose Corn Syrup—Final Rule," August 23, 1996.

25. Bray et al., "Consumption of High-Fructose Corn Syrup," 79: 537–43.

26. Sharon S. Elliott et al., "Fructose, Weight Gain, and the Insulin Resistance Syndrome," *American Journal of Clinical Nutrition,* 2002, 76, 911–922.

27. Matthias B. Schulze, JoAnn E. Manson, David S. Ludwig, Graham A. Colditz, Meir J. Stampfer, Walter C. Willett, and Frank B. Hu, "Sugar-Sweetened Beverages, Weight Gain, and Incidence of Type 2 Diabetes in Young and Middle-Aged Women," *Journal of the American Medical Association,* 2004; 292(8): 927–934.

28. Critser, *Fat Land,* 139–140. Quoting D. S. Ludwig, K. E. Peterson, and S. L. Gortmaker, "Relation Between Consumption of Sugar-Sweetened Drinks and Childhood Obesity," *Lancet,* Vol. 357, 2001, 505–508.

29. Dr. Satish Rao et al., "Fructose Intolerance: An Under-Recognized Problem," *The American Journal of Gastroenterology,* June 2003, Vol. 98, Issue 6, 1348–1353.

30. Alberto Ascherio, Meir J. Stampfer, and Walter C. Willett, "Trans Fatty Acids and Coronary Heart Disease: Background and Scientific Review," Harvard School of Public Health. Accessed March 20, 2005 at www.hsph.harvard.edu/reviews/transfats.html.

31. American Heart Association, "Heart Disease and Stroke Statistics: 2005 Update," Dallas, TX: AHA, 2005), 3.

32. Walter Willett et al., "Trans Fatty Acids and Coronary Heart Disease."

33. Walter Willett et al., referring to the Expert Panel on Trans Fatty Acids and Coronary Heart Disease, "Trans Fatty Acids and Coronary Heart Disease Risk," *American Journal of Clinical Nutrition,* 1995; 62:655S–708S. Quoted in "Trans Fatty Acids and Coronary Heart Disease."

34. Walter Willett et al., "Trans Fatty Acids and Coronary Heart Disease."

35. Carlos J. Crespo and Joshua Arbesman, "Obesity in the United States: A Worrisome Epidemic," *The Physician and Sportsmedicine,* Vol. 31, No. 11, November 2003. "The prevalence of obesity is higher among non-Hispanic black (36%) and Mexican American women (33%) than among non-Hispanic white women (22%)." See also, U.S. Centers for Disease Control, Obesity and Overweight Factsheets. Type 2 diabetes rates: G. Hosey et al., "Type 2 Diabetes in People of Color," *Nurse Practitioner Forum,* June 1998, Vol. 9, No. 2, 108–14.

36. "Median Family Income in the Past 12 Months (in 2003 inflation-adjusted dollars) by Family Size," American Community Survey, U.S. Census Bureau, 2003. Obesity rates: Shelley Hearne and Georges Benjamin, "F as in Fat: How Obesity Policies are Failing America," Trust for America's Health, October 20, 2004.

37. Foundation for Child Development, March 2005. Quoted in *USA Today,* "Obesity Weighs Down Progress in Index of Youth Well-Being," March 29, 2005. Accessed at www.usatoday.com.

38. S. Jay Olshansky, Ph.D. et al., "A Potential Decline in Life Expectancy in the United States in the 21st Century," *New England Journal of Medicine,* March 17, 2005, Vol. 352, No. 11: 1138–1145.

39. Jeffrey B. Schwimmer et al., "Health-Related Quality of Life of Severely Obese Children and Adolescents," *Journal of the American Medical Association,* April 2003; 289: 1813–1819.

40. The U.S. Centers for Disease Control and Prevention.

41. See Note 10, Chapter One, for discussion of deaths from obesity-related illnesses.

42. A. Elizabeth Sloan, "Top 10 Global Food Trends," *Food Technology,* April 2005, Vol. 59, No. 4, 21.

CHAPTER 3: ORDERING THE WAKE-UP CALL

1. Based on figures from the ETC Group. 2002 sales in U.S. dollars: seed companies: $7.1 billion; agrochemical companies: $22.3 billion; food manufacturers and traders: $259.4 billion; food retailers: $648.9 billion. Available at www.etcgroup.org.

2. Based on figures from the ETC Group. $22.3 billion in sales in 2002.

3. From *Fortune Magazine,* The 2005 Fortune 500. Available at www.fortune.com.

4. Average advertising minutes per hour on television from the American Association of Advertising Agencies. (The daytime rate was as much as 20:53 minutes per hour.) Quoted in Peter Lyman and Hal R. Varian, "How Much Information 2003?" School of Information Management and Systems, University of California at Berkeley. Accessed June 2005 at www.sims.berkeley.edu/how-much-info-2003.

5. Anthony E. Gallo, "Food Advertising in the United States," in *America's Eating Habits: Changes and Consequences,* ed. Elizabeth Frazao (Washington, D.C.: Economic Research Service, U.S. Department of Agriculture, 1999), 173–180.

6. Robert J. Coen, "Insider's Report: Robert Coen Presentation on Advertising Expenditures," McCann-Erickson Worldwide, December 2004, 8. Accessed January 26, 2005 at www.universalmccann.com/Insiders1204.pdf.

7. *Advertising Age,* "Special Report: McDonald's 50th Anniversary," July 25, 2005, S4.

8. Kelly D. Brownell and David S. Ludwig, "Fighting Obesity and the Food Lobby," *The Washington Post,* June 9, 2002, B7.

9. Clive Thompson, "There's a Sucker Born in Every Medial Prefrontal Cortex," *The New York Times Magazine,* October 26, 2003, 54.

10. Marc Graser, "McDonald's on Lookout to Be Big Mac Daddy," *Advertising Age,* March 28, 2005, 123.

11. Ibid.

12. Marian Burros, "It'd Be Easier If SpongeBob Were Hawking Broccoli," *The New York Times,* January 12, 2005, F5. See also The New Rules Project, "The Information Sector: Democratizing the Airwaves and the Wires," www.newrules.org.

13. Penny Miller, "Press Release: Soft Drinks Undermining Americans' Health: Teens Consuming Twice as Much 'Liquid Candy' as Milk," Center for Science and the Public Interest, October 21, 1998. Accessed at www.cspi.org.

14. Figures for food and beverage advertising to children from the Institute of Medicine, Committee on Prevention of Obesity in Children and Youth. See, for instance, Jeffrey P. Koplan, Catharyn T. Liverman, and Vivica A. Kraak, editors, "Preventing Childhood Obesity: Health in the Balance" (Washington, D.C., National Academies Press, 2005). Available at www.nap.edu.

15. Kaiser Family Foundation, "The Role of Media in Childhood Obesity," February 2004, The Kaiser Family Foundation, Washington, D.C. Available at www.kff.org/entmedia/entmedia022404pkg.cfm.

16. BrandWeek.com, "Food Marketers Form Ad Alliance," January 27, 2005. See also, Wendy Melillo and Aaron Baar, "Battle Lines Are Drawn Over What Makes Kids Fat," *Adweek,* January 31, 2005. Available at www.adweek.com.

17. Quoted in David Shaw, "Advertising Aimed at Kids Is Playing Hide and Seek," *Los Angeles Times,* March 6, 2005, 6.

18. Liz Marr, MS, RD, "Soft Drinks, Childhood Overweight, and the Role of Nutrition Educators: Let's Base Our Solutions on Reality and Sound Science," *Journal of Nutrition Education and Behavior,* Vol. 36, Issue 5, September 2004, 258. The article's acknowledgments state: "Funding for this article was provide by The Coca-Cola Company, Atlanta, GA." The footnote in the article also states: "Funding was provided by The Coca-Cola Company, Atlanta, GA."

19. Marian Burros, "Dental Group Is Under Fire for Coke Deal," *The New York Times,* March 4, 2003, A16. See also, Allen Kanner and Joshua Golin, "Does Coke Money Corrupt Kids' Dentists?" *Mothering,* March/April 2005, 46–51.

20. Dennis Avery, "Gulf of Mexico 'Dead Zone' Pre-Dates Farming," Center for Global Food Issues, March 7, 2005. Accessed March 15, 2005 at www.cgfi.org/materials/articles/2005/mar_07_05.htm.

21. Michael Beman, K. R. Arrigo, and P.A. Matson, "Agricultural Runoff Fuels Large Phytoplankton Blooms in Vulnerable Areas of the Ocean," *Nature,* March 10, 2005, 434: 211–214. Mark Shwartz, "Ocean Ecosystems Plagued by Agricultural Runoff," *Stanford Report,* March 16, 2005, Vol. XXXVII, No. 21, 1.

22. Author communication, Michael Beman, Stanford University, May 2005.

23. From Hudson Institute's IRS 990, year ending September 2001. Quoted at www.sourcewatch.

24. Kay Johnson, "Requiem in Orange: Decades After the U.S. Dusted Vietnam with Defoliants, Scientists and Civilians Tally the Damage," *Time Asia,* March 4, 2002. Accessed March 20, 2005 at www.time.com/time/asia/news/magazine/0,9754,214153,00.html.

25. Jon Franklin, "Poisons of the Mind," keynote address to the Society of Toxicology, March 16, 1994, quoted in Dennis Avery, *Saving the Planet with Pesticides and Plastic,* 2nd Edition (Washington, D.C.: Hudson Institute, 2000), 139.

26. Johnson, "Requiem in Orange."

27. Committee to Review the Health Effects in Vietnam Veterans of Exposure to Herbicides (Fourth Biennial Update), "Veterans and Agent Orange: Update 2002" (Washington, D.C.: Institute of Medicine, 2003). Available at www.nap.edu. See also, Christopher Marquis, "Agent Orange and Cancer Are Linked in New Study," *The New York Times,* January 24, 2003, A18.

28. William Glaberson, "In Vietnam and America, Some See a Wrong Still Not Righted," *The New York Times,* August 8, 2004, 1, 25.

29. From the National Ocean Service (NOAA). Accessed at www.nos.noaa.gov/products/pubs_hypox.html.

30. United Nations Environment Program, *Global Environment Outlook Year Book: 2004/5.* Available at www.unep.org/geo/yearbook.

31. Website registration from Network Solutions, Who Is database, March 20, 2005. *Washington University in St. Louis Magazine,* "Classmates Fall 2000," accessed March 15, 2005 at http://magazine.wustl.edu/Fall00/classmates.html.

32. Information from www.lobbywatch.org.

33. The 2001 International Consortium on Agricultural Biotechnology Conference program, accessible at www.economia.uniroma2.it/conferenze/icabr01/Program.htm.

34. Jonathan Matthews, "Biotech's Hall of Mirrors: From Berkeley to Johannesburg, from India to Zambia, Biotech's Deceivers Are Playing a Very Dirty Game," GeneWatch, Vol. 16, No. 1, January–February 2003. Available at www.genewatch.org.

35. David Quist and Ignacio H. Chapela, "Transgenic DNA Introgressed into Traditional Maize Landraces in Oaxaca, Mexico," *Nature,* November 29, 2001, 414, 541–543. See also, George Monbiot, "The Covert Biotech War," *The Guardian,* November 19, 2002. Accessed at www.guardian.co.uk.

36. See, for instance, Claire Hope Cummings, "Trespass," *World Watch,* January/February 2005. Available at www.worldwatch.org.

37. George Monbiot, "The Fake Persuaders," *The Guardian* (UK), May 14, 2002. Accessed March 2005 at www.guardian.co.uk/comment/story/0,3604,715153,00.html.

38. Ibid.

39. Ibid.

40. Author communication, Alex Knott, Center for Public Integrity, June 2005. Lobbying spending increased nearly 50 percent, from $1.4 billion in 1998 to $2.1 billion in 2004.

41. Author communication, Alex Knott, Center for Public Integrity, June 2005. The Center looked at six years of reporting and found 20 percent of lobbying forms were filed late, and an additional 20 percent were never filed at all.

42. Data from the Center for Responsive Politics, www.opensecrets.org.

43. Associated Press, "House Passes $180B Farm Bill," May 2, 2002.

44. Data from the Center for Public Integrity's Lobbywatch. Available at www.publicintegrity.org.

45. Data from U.S. Office of Public Records Lobby Filing Disclosure Program. Available at http://sopr.senate.gov/.

46. Data from the Center for Public Integrity's Lobbywatch. Available at www.publicintegrity.org.

47. Bill Summary and Status for the 108th Congress. Viewed March 20, 2005 at http://thomas.loc.gov/cgi-bin/bdquery/z?d108:h.r.04651.

48. From the Grocery Manufacturers of America, www.gmabrands.com. Data from 1997 to 2000 on www.opensecrets.org. Data from 2000 to 2004 from the U.S. Office of Public Records Lobby Filing Disclosure Program: http://sopr.senate.gov/.

49. Data from the Center for Public Integrity's Lobbywatch. Available at www.publicintegrity.org. GMA reported $1.22 million for lobbying in 2004.

50. From the Grocery Manufacturers of America, Policy Briefs. Available at www.gmabrands.com.

51. Ibid.

52. From the Oklahoma Fit Kids Coalition. Accessed at www.integrislifespan.com.

53. Letter to Stephen Johnson at U.S. EPA Headquarters, from Jay Vroom, President CropLife America, and Allen James, President, RISE. Re: NEETF Forum "National Strategies for Health Care Providers: Pesticide Initiative," July 8, 2002.

54. Letter referring to panels listed on the National Forum Draft Agenda, "National Strategies for Health Care Providers: Pesticide Initiative," September 19–20, 2002.

55. From www.sourcewatch.org.

56. National Environmental Education and Training Foundation, National Strategies for Health Care Providers, Pesticides Initiative, Proceedings for the June 10–11, 2003 National Forum. Appendix A, National Forum Agenda, and Appendix B, Speaker Presentations.

57. Dan Fagin, Marianne Lavelle, and the Center for Public Integrity, *Toxic Deception: How the Chemical Industry Manipulates Science, Bends the Law, and Endangers Your Health* (Secaucus, NJ: Birch Lane Publishing, 1996), xi.

58. Ibid.

59. Elizabeth Brown, "More Than 2,000 Spin Through Revolving Door," April 7, 2005. From the Center for Public Integrity, available at www.publicintegrity.org.

60. For more information, visit the Edmonds Institute, Revolving Door Database: www.edmonds-institute.org/door.html. See also, the "Top Revolvers" at the Center for Public Integrity's Reporter Tools: www.publicintegrity.org. See also, Skip Spitzer, "Industrial Agriculture and Corporate Power," *Global Pesticide Campaigner* Vol. 13, No. 2, August 31, 2003, 1, 12–15.

61. Philip Mattera, "USDA Inc.: How Agribusiness Has Hijacked Regulatory Policy at the U.S. Department of Agriculture" (Washington, D.C.: Agribusiness Accountability Initiative and the Corporate Research Project of Good Jobs First), July 23, 2004, 28.

62. The policy council was the International Policy Council on Agriculture, Food and Trade. For more information, see *USDA Inc.*

63. BIO 2005 Annual Convention press release. Available at www.bio.org.

64. See Claire Hope Cummings, "Trespass," *World Watch,* January/February 2005, 24–35. Available at www.worldwatch.org.

65. See, for example, the forum "The Pulse of Scientific Freedom in the Age of the Biotech Industry," UC Berkeley, December 2003. Available at http://nature.berkeley.edu/pulseofscience/pix/conv.txt1.html. Quoted in Cummings, "Trespass," 34.

66. See Melody Petersen, "Farmers' Right to Sue Grows, Raising Debate on Food Safety," *The New York Times,* June 1, 1999, A1.

67. See, for example, Irving Janis, *Victims of Groupthink: A Psychological Study of Foreign-Policy Decisions and Fiascoes* (Boston, MA: Houghton Mifflin, 1972), and Irving Janis and Leon Mann, *Decision Making: A Psychological Analysis of Conflict, Choice and Commitment* (New York: The Free Press, 1977).

CHAPTER 4: GRUB 101

1. Concern about pesticides: Natural Marketing Institute data, posted on *PR Newswire,* April 12, 2005. Organic consumption trends: author communication, Holly Givens, Communications Director, Organic Trade Association, April 2005.

2. Roughly three-quarters of all conventional grocery stores nationwide now carry organic foods according to a 2002 Food Marketing Institute study.

3. Donald W. Lotter, "Organic Agriculture," *Journal of Sustainable Agriculture,* Vol. 21, Issue 4 2003, 59–128.

4. Latest available figures. From USDA, Economic Research Service.

5. Author communication, Catherine Greene, ERS. See also, Market Profile of Organic Goods, www.fas.usda.gov/agx/organics/news.htm.

6. USDA, Economic Research Service. Accessed at www.ers.usda.gov/StateFacts/US.htm.

7. International Federation of Organic Agriculture Movements, "The World of Organic Agriculture: Statistics and Emerging Trends 2005," June 2005. Available at www.ifoam.org.

8. Ibid.

9. Norman Uphoff, ed., *Agroecological Innovations: Increasing Food Production with Participatory Development* (London, Earthscan: 2001). See, for example, "Chapter 11: Increasing Productivity through Agroecological Approaches in Central America: Experiences from Hillside Agriculture."

10. Jules Pretty and Rachel Hine, "Reducing Food Poverty with Sustainable Agriculture," Center for Environment and Society, University of Essex, UK, February, 2001. Available at http://www2.essex.ac.uk/ces/ ResearchProgrammes/SAFEWexecsummfinalreport.htm.

11. David Pimentel et al., "Environmental, Energetic, and Economic Comparisons of Organic and Conventional Farming Systems," *Bioscience,* July 2005, Vol. 55, No. 7, 573–582(10).

12. Ibid.

13. Uphoff, ed., *Agroecological Innovations.* See, for example, "Chapter 1: Can a More Agroecological Agriculture Feed a Growing World Population?"

14. Based on research by Dr. Charles Benbrook, former executive director of the board on agriculture at the National Academy of Sciences, examining 10,000 field trials of GMO soybeans over four years. Dr. Charles M. Benbrook, "Troubled Times Amid Commercial Success for Roundup Ready Soybeans Glyphosate Efficacy Is Slipping and Unstable Transgene Expression Erodes Plant Defenses and Yields," BioTech InfoNet, Technical Paper Number 4, May 3, 2001. Available at www.biotech-info.net.

15. Dr. Charles M. Benbrook, "Genetically Engineered Crops and Pesticide Use in the United States: The First Nine Years," BioTech InfoNet, Technical Paper Number 7, October 2004, 2. Available at www.biotech-info.net.

16. Author communication, Ronnie Cummins, Organic Consumers Association. June 2005.

17. Ibid.

18. USDA and Health and Human Services, "Dietary Guidelines for Americans," January 12, 2005. The Dietary Guidelines has been published jointly every five years since 1980 by HHS and the USDA. Viewable at www .health.gov/dietaryguidelines/.

19. Joan Gussow, quoted in *Organic Gardening,* September/October 2002, 39.

20. Food Circles Networking Project, "The Guide to Eating Well and Doing Good in Columbia, Missouri" (Columbia, MO: University of Missouri Extension, 2005). Available at www.foodcircles.missouri.edu.

21. Author communication, Professor Mike Hamm, May 2005.

22. Kamyar Enshayan, "Local Food Purchases by Institutional Food Buyers in Black Hawk and Surrounding Counties, Iowa 2004," University of Northern Iowa Local Food Project, Cedar Falls, Iowa.

23. "Price-Tag/Cost-Tag," Center for Integrated Agricultural Systems, College of Agricultural and Life Sciences, UW–Madison, 2003.

24. Estimates from the Department of Labor, "Pesticides: Improvements Needed to Ensure the Safety of Farmworkers and Their Children," Government Accountability Office, Report to Congressional Requesters, GAO/RCED-00-40, March 2000, 6.

25. National Agricultural Worker Survey 2000. The most reliable figures are from the national survey conducted by U.S. Department of Labor until 2005, when the survey was suspended as a result of budget cuts. Miriam

Jordan, "Labor Department Ends Survey of Migrant Farm-Worker Status," *The Wall Street Journal,* January 24, 2005, A4.

26. National Agricultural Worker Survey 2000. Based on Bureau of Labor statistics of fatalities and non-fatal injuries.

27. Human Rights Watch, Children's Rights Project. Available at www.hri.ca/children/.

28. From the Department of Labor, "Pesticides: Improvements Needed," 17.

29. Human Rights Watch, "Fingers to the Bone: United States Failure to Protect Child Farmworkers" (New York: Human Rights Watch), June 2000.

30. From the Department of Labor, "Pesticides: Improvements Needed," 6.

31. John Lantigua and Christine Stapleton, "Pesticide Use Data: Florida Pesticide Monitoring Draws Fire," *Palm Beach Post,* April 25, 2005. Accessed at www.palmbeachpost.com.

32. Janine A. Zeitlin, "State Probing Possible Birth Defect Link Among Farmworkers' Babies," *Naples Daily News,* March 15, 2005. Accessed at www.naplesnews.com.

33. From the Department of Labor, "Pesticides: Improvements Needed," 22.

34. Margaret Reeves, Anne Katten, and Martha Guzmán, "Fields of Poison 2002: California Farmworkers and Pesticides" (San Francisco, CA: Pesticide Action Network of North America, 2002).

35. Hannah Sassaman, "Farmworkers Win a Penny More," *YES! A Journal of Positive Futures,* Summer 2005, 9.

36. Associated Press, "First, They Took on Taco Bell. Now, the Fast-Food World," *The New York Times,* May 22, 2005, A25.

37. Author communication, Heather Franzese, TransFair USA, December 2004.

CHAPTER 5: HEALTH 411

1. The Fertilizer Institute, *Setting the Record Straight* DVD, September 2003. Available at www.tfi.org.

2. CropLife International, promotional materials, December 20, 2000.

3. André Picard, "Organic Crops No More Nutritional," *The Globe and Mail,* July 8, 2002, A1.

4. Ibid., A7.

5. From Guelph University's Food Safety Network's online list of donors. Accessed March 29, 2005 at www .foodsafetynetwork.ca/funding.htm.

6. Charles M. Benbrook, Ph.D., "Elevating Antioxidant Levels in Food Through Organic Farming and Food Processing," An Organic Center State of Science Review, January 2005, 22. Available at www.organic-center .org.

7. Marian Burros, "Eating Well: Is Organic Food Probably Better?" *The New York Times,* July 16, 2003, F1.

8. Danny K. Asami, Yun-Jeong Hong, Diane M. Barrett, and Alyson E. Mitchell, "Comparison of the Total Phenolic and Ascorbic Acid Content of Freeze-Dried and Air-Dried Marionberry, Strawberry, and Corn Grown Using Conventional, Organic, and Sustainable Agricultural Practices," *Journal of Agricultural and Food Chemistry,* February 2003, 26; Vol. 51, No. 5, 1237–41.

9. H. Ren, H. Endo, and T. Hayashi, "Antioxidative and Antimutagenic Activities and Polyphenol Content of Pesticide-Free and Organically-Cultivated Green Vegetables Using Water-Soluble Chiosan as a Soil Modifier and Leaf Surface Spray," *Journal of the Science of Food and Agriculture*, 2001, Vol. 81, No. 15, 1426–1432.

10. From Charles M. Benbrook, Ph.D., "Elevating Antioxidant Levels," quoting Lisbeth Grinder-Pedersen, Salka E. Rasmussen, Susanne Bügel, Lars V. Jørgensen, Lars O. Dragsted, Vagn Gundersen, and Brittmarie Sandström, "Effect of Diets Based on Foods from Conventional versus Organic Production on Intake and Excretion of Flavonoids and Markers of Antioxidative Defense in Humans," *Journal of Agricultural and Food Chemistry*, 2003, Vol. 51, No. 19, 5671.

11. Ibid.

12. See, for example, Marina Carbonaro, Maria Mattera, Stefano Nicoli, Paolo Bergamo, and Marsilio Cappelloni, "Modulation of Antioxidant Compounds in Organic vs. Conventional Fruit (peach, Prunus persica L., and pear, Pyrus communis L.)," *Journal of Agricultural and Food Chemistry*, September 2002, Vol. 50, No. 19, 5458–62.

13. J. F. Tomera, "Current Knowledge of the Health Benefits and Disadvantages of Wine Consumption," *Trends in Food Science and Technology*, April 1999, Vol. 10, No. 4, 129–138.

14. Henry Brockman, *Organic Matters* (Congerville, IL: Terra Books, 2001), 9. Available at www.theland connection.org.

15. Ibid., 16.

16. Ibid., 18.

17. Benbrook, "Elevating Antioxidant Levels."

18. Transcript of organic food safety report, ABC News *20/20*, Feb. 4, 2000, "How Good Is Organic Food? *20/20*'s John Stossel Investigates." Accessed March 29, 2005 at www.cgfi.org/materials/articles/2000/sep_29_00.htm.

19. Ibid.

20. Transcript posted on www.ewg.org/reports/givemeafake/transcript.html.

21. Donald W. Lotter, "Organic Agriculture," 23.

22. Dennis Avery, "Clusters/Outbreaks of *E. coli* O157:H7 reported to CDC in 1996," *American Outlook*, Hudson Institute, 1998. Available at www.cfgi.org.

23. Stossel's retraction available at "Chronology of John Stossel's Flawed Organic Food Story," accessed March 29, 2005 at www.ewg.org/reports/givemeafake/newdevelopments.html. See also, Dr. Mitchell Cohen, CDC, statement from January 1999: "*E. coli* and the Safety of Organic Food."

24. Dennis Avery data available at www.cgfi.org/materials/articles/1999/feb_27_99.htm#table.

25. The Soil Association, "*E. coli* and the Safety of Organic Food," accessed April 5, 2005 at www.soilassociation.org/web/sa/saweb.nsf/librarytitles/Briefing_Sheets30091999.

26. CNN, "E. Coli Poisoning Leads to Odwalla Juice Recall," November 1, 1996. Accessed March 29, 2005 at www.cnn.com/HEALTH/9611/01/e.coli.poisoning/.

27. Owen McShane, "Straight Thinking: Organics Good, Genetically Modified Bad. Yeah, Right," *The National Business Review* (New Zealand), August 6, 2004, 29.

28. Author communication, Owen McShane, November 2004.

29. Sonja J. Olsen, Ph.D., Linda C. MacKinon, MPH, Joy S. Goulding, Nancy H. Bean, Ph.D., and Laurence Slutsker, MD, "Surveillance for Foodborne Disease Outbreaks—United States, 1993–1997, "Division of Bacterial and Mycotic Diseases, National Center for Infectious Diseases, March 17, 2000, 49(SS01); 1–51.

30. Most recent data available: Paul Mead et al., "Food-Related Illness and Death in the United States," Centers for Disease Control, Atlanta, Georgia, 1999. Available at www.cdc.gov/ncidod/eid/vol5no5/mead.htm. Totals are an estimate of known and unknown pathogens; known pathogens accounted for 14 million illnesses, 60,000 hospitalizations, and 1,800 deaths.

31. National Institutes of Health, U.S. Department of Health and Human Services, Fact Sheets, February 2005, www.niaid.nih.gov/factsheets/foodbornedis.htm.

32. The Centers for Disease Control and Prevention estimates that 73,000 cases of *E. coli* O157:H7 occur every year in the United States. 2,100 people are hospitalized, and 61 people die as a direct result of *E. coli* infections and complications that can result from infections. Accessed April 5, 2005, www.cdc.gov/ncidod/dbmd/diseaseinfo/escherichiacoli_t.htm.

33. National Institutes of Health, U.S. Department of Health and Human Services, "Foodborne Illnesses," February 2005. Accessed April 5, 2005 at www.niaid.nih.gov/factsheets/foodbornedis.htm.

34. Marion Nestle, *Safe Food: Bacteria, Biotechnology, and Bioterrorism* (Berkeley, CA: University of California Press, 2003), 45. See especially "Chapter 1: The Politics of Foodborne Illness."

35. Cook, *Diet for a Dead Planet,* 60.

36. Ibid., 63.

37. Associated Press, "Bacteria Fears Prompt Largest Ever U.S. Meat Recall," October 14, 2002. (Serving size based on USDA recommendations.)

38. USDA and FDA recalls data available at www.recalls.gov.

39. Avery, *Saving the Planet with Pesticides and Plastic,* 69.

40. Ibid., 13.

41. Solomon et al., *Generations at Risk,* 120.

42. See, for example, Julie L. Daniels et al., "Pesticides and Childhood Cancers," *Environmental Health Perspectives,* October 1997, Vol. 105, No. 10, 1068–1077; Janice M. Pogoda and Susan Preston-Martin, "Household Pesticides and Risk of Pediatric Brain Tumors," *Environmental Health Perspectives,* November 1997, Vol. 105, No. 11, 1214–1220; James R. Davis et al., "Family Pesticide Use and Childhood Brain Cancer," *Archives of Environmental Contamination and Toxicology,* 1993, Vol. 24, 87–92.

43. Dick Taverne, "A Little Pesticide Does You Good But 'Organic' Farming Harms the World," *The Sunday Telegraph* (UK), March 13, 2005. (Adapted from Dick Taverne, *The March of Unreason: Science, Democracy, and the New Fundamentalism* [Oxford University Press, 2005]).

44. See, for example, A. Blair et al., "Mortality Among Participants in the Agricultural Health Study," *Annals of Epidemiology,* Vol. 15, Issue 4, 279–285.

45. Avery, *Saving the Planet with Pesticides and Plastic,* 13.

46. Brian P. Baker, Charles M. Benbrook, Edward Groth III, and Karen Lutz Benbrook, "Pesticide Residues in Conventional, IPM-Grown and Organic Foods: Insights from Three U.S. Data Sets," *Food Additives and Contaminants,* Vol. 19, No. 5, May, 2002, 427–446. See also, "Greener Greens? The Truth about Organic Foods," *Consumer Reports,* January 1998, 13; and Edward Groth III, "Do You Know What You're Eating? An Analysis of U.S. Government Data on Pesticide Residues in Foods," *Consumers Union,* February 1999. Available at www.consumersunion.org.

47. See, for example, "Chemical Trespass: Pesticides in Our Bodies and Corporate Accountability" (San Francisco, CA: Pesticide Action Network of North America, 2004). Available at www.panna.org.

48. Wargo, *Our Children's Toxic Legacy,* 114.

49. Cynthia L. Curl, Richard A. Fenske, Kai Elgethun, "Organophosphorus Pesticide Exposure of Urban and Suburban Preschool Children with Organic and Conventional Diets," Department of Environmental Health, School of Public Health and Community Medicine, University of Washington, Seattle, *Environmental Health Perspectives,* March 2003, 111(3): 377–82. See also, Hestien J. I. Vreugdenhil, Froukje M. E. Slijper, Paul G. H. Mulder, and Nynke Weisglas-Kuperus, "Effects of Perinatal Exposure to PCBs and Dioxins on Play Behavior in Dutch Children at School Age," *Environmental Health Perspectives,* October 2002, 110(10): A593–8.

50. Wargo, *Our Children's Toxic Legacy,* 4.

51. From an analysis of U.S. customs records by Carl Smith, "Pesticide Exports from U.S. Ports, 1997–2000," *International Journal of Occupational and Environmental Health,* October–December 2001, Vol. 7, No. 4, 266–74.

52. See, for example, David Weir and Mark Schapiro, *Circle of Poison: Pesticides and People in a Hungry World* (Oakland, CA: Food First, 1981).

53. See, for example, Institute for Agriculture and Trade Policy, Food and Health Issue areas, available at www.iatp.org.

CHAPTER 6: SEVEN STEPS TO A GRUB KITCHEN

1. Data from Take Back Your Time Day, a U.S./Canadian initiative to challenge the epidemic of overwork, overscheduling and "time famine" that now threatens our health, our families and relationships, our communities and our environment. Learn more at www.timeday.org.

2. Jayachandran N. Variyam, "Nutrition Labeling in the Food-Away-From-Home Sector: An Economic Assessment," USDA Economic Research Service, April 2005. Americans spent about 46 percent of their total food budget on food away from home in 2002, up from 27 percent in 1962.

3. Author communication, Timothy Jones, University of Arizona, March 2005.

4. USDA, Economic Research Service.

5. Thomas A. Lyson, *Civic Agriculture: Reconnecting Farm, Food, and Community* (Lebanon, NH: Tufts University Press, 2004), 91.

6. For more information: ams.usda.gov/farmersmarkets/FMstudystats.htm.

7. Community Food Security Coalition, North American Urban Agriculture Committee, "Urban Agriculture and Community Food Security in the United States: Farming from the City Center to the Urban Fringe," October 2003. Available at www.foodsecurity.org.

8. Ibid.

9. Author communication, Betsy Johnson, Interim Director, American Community Gardening Association, January 2005.

10. See also Frances Cerra Whittelsey, "Hazards of Hydration: Choose Your Plastic Water Bottles Carefully," *Sierra Magazine,* viewed at sierraclub.org/sierra/200311/lol5.asp. Theo Colborn, John Peterson Myers, and Dianne Dumanoski, *Our Stolen Future* (New York: Plume Books, 1997), 215.

11. U.S. Geological Survey, "Pharmaceuticals, Hormones, and Other Organic Wastewater Contaminants in U.S. Streams," USGS Fact Sheet FS-027-02, June 2002.

12. Jeremiah Baumann, Sean Gray, Jane Houlihan, and Richard Wiles, "Consider the Source: Farm Runoff, Chlorination Byproducts, and Human Health" (Washington, D.C.: Environmental Working Group and the State PIRGS, 2002), 1. Available at www.ewg.org.

13. See, for example, Erik D. Olson, "Bottled Water: Pure Drink or Pure Hype?" (Washington, D.C.: Natural Resources Defense Council, February 1999). Available at www.nrdc.org.

14. Colborn et al., *Our Stolen Future,* 217.

15. See, for example, Margaret Sanborn et al., "Systematic Review of Pesticide Human Health Effects," Ontario College of Family Physicians in Canada (Toronto, Canada), April 23, 2004. Accessible at www.ocfp.on.ca/english/ocfp/default.asp?s=1.

16. "The Grass Crop of the Chesapeake Bay Watershed," *Envirocast Weather & Watershed Newsletter,* Vol. 1, No. 7, National Environmental Education and Training Foundation and the Center for Watershed Protection, May 2003. Average pesticide usage on farmland: Robert Kellogg, Richard Nehring, Art Grube, et al., "Trends in the Potential for Environmental Risk from Pesticide Loss from Farm Fields," EPA and USDA, Presentation for "The State of North America's Private Land" conference, Chicago, IL, January 19–21, 1999.

17. Pesticide usage on golf courses: Mark Wexler, "Travel Column: Greener Golf Is Growing—Slowly," *National Geographic Traveler,* June 25, 2004.

18. E. Michael Thurman, Lisa R. Zimmerman, Elisabeth A. Scribner, and Richard H. Coupe Jr., "Occurrence of Cotton Pesticides in Surface Water of the Mississippi Embayment, USGS Fact Sheet 022–98, May 1998. Accessed April 14, 2005.

19. Environmental Working Group, "Skin Deep," Washington, D.C., June 2004. Available at www.ewg.org.

CHAPTER 7: OUT OF THE KITCHEN, INTO THE FIRE

1. Rachel Carson, *Silent Spring* (Boston, MA: Houghton Mifflin, 1962), 277.

2. Figures from Technomic, Inc. 2004–2005 U.S. "Foodservice Industry Forecast," Food purchases at college and universities amounted to $4.398 billion.

3. Author communication, Kristen Markley, National Farm-to-College Program Manager, Community Food Security Coalition, May 2005.

4. Author communication, Marion Kalb, Farm-to-School coordinator, Community Food Security Coalition, February 2005.

5. Data from Food and Nutrition Service, USDA, www.fns.usda.gov.

6. Author communication, David Leggett, Department of Defense Fresh Fruit and Vegetable Program, July 2005.

7. Mike Geniella, "Ruling Lets Language of Mendocino County Ballot Measure Stand for March 2 Election," *The Press Democrat*, December 31, 2003.

8. Author communication, Britt Bailey, Environmental Commons, June 2005.

Bibliography

Ackerman, Frank, and Lisa Heinzerling. *Priceless: On Knowing the Price of Everything and the Value of Nothing.* New York: The New Press, 2004.

Ausubel, Kenny, and J. P. Harpignies. *Nature's Operating Instructions: The True Biotechnologies.* San Francisco: Sierra Club Books, 2004.

Avery, Dennis. *Saving the Planet with Pesticides and Plastic: The Environmental Triumph of High-Yield Farming, 2nd Ed.* Indianapolis, IN: Hudson Institute, 2000.

Balfour, Eve B. *The Living Soil and the Haughley Experiment.* London: Faber & Faber, 1943.

Barstow, Cynthia. *Eco-Foods Guide: What's Good for the Earth Is Good for You!* St. Paul, MN: Consortium, 2002.

Berley, Peter. *The Modern Vegetarian Kitchen.* New York: Regan Books, 2000.

Berry, Wendell. *The Unsettling of America: Culture and Agriculture.* San Francisco: Sierra Club Books, 1977.

Brownell, Kelly D., and Katherine Battle Horgen. *Food Fight: The Inside Story of the Food Industry, America's Obesity Crisis, and What We Can Do About It.* New York: McGraw-Hill, 2003.

Brush, Stephen B. *Farmers' Bounty: Locating Crop Diversity in the Contemporary World.* New Haven, CT: Yale University Press, 2004.

Carson, Rachel. *Silent Spring.* Minneapolis: Sagebrush, 2002. Original publication date: 1962.

Chaskey, Scott. *This Common Ground: Seasons on an Organic Farm.* New York: Viking Press, 2005.

Colbin, Annemarie. *Food and Healing.* New York: Ballantine Books, 1986.

Colborn, Theo, John Peterson Myers, and Dianne Dumanoski. *Our Stolen Future: Are We Threatening Our Own Fertility, Intelligence, and Survival?—A Scientific Detective Story.* New York: Plume Books, 1997.

Cook, Christopher D. *Diet for a Dead Planet: How the Food Industry Is Killing Us.* New York: The New Press, 2004.

Cool, Jesse Ziff. *Your Organic Kitchen: Essential Guide to Selecting and Cooking Organic Foods.* Emmaus, PA: Rodale Books, 2002.

Cooper, Ann, and Lisa M. Holmes. *Bitter Harvest: A Chef's Perspective on the Hidden Danger in the Foods We Eat and What We Can Do About It.* New York: Routledge, 2000.

Critser, Greg. *Fat Land: How Americans Became the Fattest People in the World.* New York: Houghton Mifflin, 2003.

Cummins, Ronnie, and Ben Lilliston. *Genetically Engineered Food: A Self-Defense Guide for Consumers.* Berkeley, CA: Marlowe & Company, 2000.

Fagin, Dan, Marianne Lavelle, and the Center for Public Integrity. *Toxic Deception: How the Chemical Industry Manipulates Science, Bends the Law, and Endangers Your Health.* Monroe, ME: Common Courage Press, 1999.

Fernandez-Armesto, Felipe. *Food: A History.* London: Pan Macmillan, 2002.

Galeano, Eduardo. *Upside Down World.* New York: Picador, 2001.

Gregory, Dick. *Dick Gregory's Natural Diet for Folks Who Eat: Cookin' with Mother Nature.* Ed. James R. McGraw and Alvenia M. Fulton. New York: Perennial Library, 1973.

Gussow, Joan. *This Organic Life: Confessions of a Suburban Homesteader.* White River Junction, VT: Chelsea Green, 2002.

Guthman, Julie. *Agrarian Dreams.* Berkeley, CA: University of California Press, 2004.

Halweil, Brian. *Eat Here: Homegrown Pleasures in a Global Supermarket.* New York: W. W. Norton & Company, 2004.

Hines, Colin. *Localization: A Global Manifesto.* London: Earthscan, 2000.

Jamieson, Alex. *The Great American Detox Diet: The Proven 8-Week Program for Weight Loss, Good Health and Well Being.* Emmaus, PA: Rodale Books, 2005.

Jasanoff, Sheila. *The Fifth Branch: Science Advisors as Policymakers.* Cambridge, MA: Harvard University Press, 1990.

Katzen, Mollie. *The New Moosewood Cookbook.* Berkeley, CA: Ten Speed Press, 2000.

Kimbrell, Andrew, ed. *Fatal Harvest: The Tragedy of Industrial Agriculture.* Washington, D.C.: Island Press, 2002.

Krimsky, Sheldon. *Hormonal Chaos: The Scientific and Social Origins of the Environmental Endocrine Hypothesis.* Baltimore: Johns Hopkins Press, 2002.

Landrigan, Philip, J., Herbert Needleman, and Mary Landrigan. *Raising Healthy Children in a Toxic World: 101 Smart Solutions for Every Family.* Emmaus, PA: Rodale Press, 2002.

Lappé, Frances Moore. *Diet for a Small Planet (20th Anniversary ed.).* New York: Ballantine Books, 1991.

Lappé, Frances Moore, and Anna Lappé. *Hope's Edge: The Next Diet for a Small Planet.* New York: Jeremy P. Tarcher/Putnam, 2002.

Lappé, Frances Moore, and Joseph Collins. *Food First.* New York: Ballantine Books, 1981.

Lappé, Frances Moore, Joseph Collins, Peter Rosset, and the Institute for Food and Development Policy. *World Hunger: Twelve Myths.* Berkeley, CA: Grove Press, 1999.

Lappé, Marc. *Germs That Won't Die: Medical Consequences of the Misuse of Antibiotics.* Garden City, NY: Anchor Books, 1982.

———. *When Antibiotics Fail: Restoring the Ecology of the Body.* Berkeley, CA: North Atlantic Books, 1986.

Lappé, Marc, and Britt Bailey. *Against the Grain: Biotechnology and the Corporate Takeover of Your Food.* Monroe, ME: Common Courage Press, 1998.

Lipson, Elaine Marie. *The Organic Foods Sourcebook.* New York: Contemporary Books, 2001.

Lyson, Thomas A. *Civic Agriculture: Reconnecting Farm, Food, and Community.* Lebanon, NH: Tufts University Press, 2004.

McEarhern, Leslie, and John Begelow Taylor. *The Angelica Home Kitchen: Recipes and Rabble Rousings from an Organic Vegan Restaurant.* Berkeley, CA: Ten Speed Press, 2003.

National Academy of Sciences. *Pesticides in the Diets of Infants and Children.* Washington, D.C.: National Academy Press, 1993.

Nestle, Marion. *Food Politics: How the Food Industry Influences Nutrition and Health.* Berkeley, CA: University of California Press, 2003.

———. *Safe Food: Bacteria, Biotechnology, and Bioterrorism.* Berkeley, CA: University of California Press, 2003.

———. *What to Eat.* New York: Farrar, Straus, & Giroux, 2006.

Onstad, Dianne. *Whole Foods Companion: A Guide for Adventurous Cooks, Curious Shoppers, and Lovers of Natural Foods.* White River Junction, VT: Chelsea Green, 1996.

Robbins, John. *The Food Revolution: How Your Diet Can Help Save Your Life and Our World.* York Beach, ME: Conari Press, 2001.

Salatin, Joel. *Holy Cows and Hog Heaven: The Food Buyer's Guide to Farm Friendly Food.* White River Junction, VT: Chelsea Green, 2004.

Schettler, Ted, Gina Solomon, Maria Valenti, and Annette Huddle. *Generations at Risk: Reproductive Health and the Environment.* Cambridge, MA: MIT Press, 2000.

Schlosser, Eric. *Fast Food Nation: The Dark Side of the All-American Meal.* New York: Houghton Mifflin, 2001.

———. *Reefer Madness: Sex, Drugs, and Cheap Labor in the American Black Market.* New York: Houghton Mifflin, 2001.

Shiva, Vandana. *Monocultures of the Mind: Perspectives on Biodiversity and Biotechnology.* London: Zed Books, 1993.

———. *Stolen Harvest: The Hijacking of the Global Food Supply.* Cambridge, MA: South End Press, 2000.

Shuman, Michael. *Going Local: Creating Self-Reliant Communities in a Global Age.* New York: The Free Press, 1998.

Smith, Jeffrey M. *Genetic Roulette: The Documented Health Risks of Genetically Engineered Foods.* Fairfield, IA: Yes! Books, 2005.

———. *Seeds of Deception: Exposing Industry and Government Lies about the Safety of the Genetically Engineered Foods That You're Eating.* Fairfield, IA: Yes! Books, 2003.

Stauber, John, and Sheldon Rampton. *Mad Cow USA.* Monroe, ME: Common Courage Press, 1997.

———. *Toxic Sludge Is Good for You: Lies, Damn Lies and the Public Relations Industry.* Monroe, ME: Common Courage Press, 1995.

———. *Trust Us, We're Experts: How Industry Manipulates Science and Gambles with Your Future.* New York: Penguin Putnam, 2002.

Steingraber, Sandra. *Living Downstream.* New York: Addison-Wesley, 1997.

Thompson, Charles, and Melinda Wiggins. *The Human Cost of Food: Farmworkers' Lives, Labor, and Advocacy.* Austin, TX: University of Texas, Austin, 2002.

Van den Bosch, Robert. *The Pesticide Conspiracy.* Berkeley, CA: University of California Press, 1989.

Willett, Walter, and P. J. Skerrett. *Eat, Drink, and Be Healthy: The Harvard Medical School Guide to Healthy Eating.* New York: The Free Press, 2002.

Wargo, John. *Our Children's Toxic Legacy: How Science and Law Fail to Protect Us from Pesticides.* New Haven, CT: Yale University Press, Second Edition, 1998.

Wood, Rebecca. *The New Whole Foods Encyclopedia: A Comprehensive Resource for Healthy Eating.* New York: Penguin, 1999.

About the Authors

ANNA LAPPÉ

Anna Lappé began developing her interest in food at the ripe age of three, when she accompanied her mother on a research trip to Guatemala. Since then, she's lived and worked in South Africa, France, and England and has traveled to more than twenty-five countries, most recently in researching her first book, *Hope's Edge*. Coauthored with her mother, Frances Moore Lappé, the nationally bestselling *Hope's Edge* chronicles courageous social movements around the world, including Nobel Peace Laureate Wangari Maathai's Green Belt Movement.

With Frances Moore Lappé, Anna leads the Cambridge, Massachusetts–based Small Planet Institute, a collaborative network for research and popular education. Founded in 2004, the Institute has produced several books, numerous articles, and various media tools for activists. Anna is also the cofounder of the volunteer-led Small Planet Fund, which supports grassroots changemakers around the world addressing the root causes of hunger and poverty.

Anna lectures extensively about food politics, democracy, and healthy communities, speaking to audiences from Columbia graduate students to Long Island high schoolkids and octogenarian Unitarians. Anna is also a big believer in the power of film and is working with Sierra Club Productions on a documentary based on *Hope's Edge*.

Anna holds an M.A. in economic and political development from Columbia University's School of International and Public Affairs and a B.A. with honors from Brown University, but believes most of her best learning has happened outside the classroom walls.

She is currently a Food and Society Policy Fellow, a national program of the WK Kellogg Foundation, and lives in Brooklyn, where sometimes—when she's lucky—Bryant comes to visit.

BRYANT TERRY

Bryant's passion for Grub can be traced back to his childhood in Memphis, Tennessee, where his grandparents inspired him to grow, cook, and appreciate food. Over the past five years, he has committed himself to feeding people and illuminating the connections between poverty, malnutrition, and institutional racism.

In 2001, Bryant founded b-healthy! (Build Healthy Eating and Lifestyles to Help Youth), a New York City–based not-for-profit organization made up of adult and youth social justice activists, chefs, and mothers working to strengthen the food justice movement in the United States and beyond.

Bryant is nationally recognized for his persistent effort to innovatively create a more just and sustainable food system, and he has received numerous awards for his work, which include an Open Society Institute Community Fellowship (Soros Foundation), a Wave of the Future Award (Glynwood Center), and a Sea Change Residency (Gaea Foundation).

As a whole foods chef, Bryant caters events—from small business meetings to week-long activist retreats—providing delicious, health-supportive food and education about the personal and environmental benefits of maintaining a healthy diet. Because his family surrounded him with literature, music, and visual art, in addition to cooking, Bryant expresses himself through creative writing, deejaying, photography, and collage. His words and images have appeared in numerous publications.

Bryant graduated from the chef's training program at the Natural Gourmet Cookery School in New York City. He holds an M.A. in history from New York University and a B.A. with honors in English from Xavier University of Louisiana.

He lives in Oakland and frequently returns to The Planet—Brooklyn, that is.

EatGrub.org

We created eatgrub.org as a complement to this book, providing additional resources and learning tools, including shopping lists and playlists for Grub menus. The site also links you to the incredible organizations around the world bringing Grub to life and offers ideas for hosting your own Grub parties.

See you online!

ANNA LAPPÉ AND BRYANT TERRY

The Grub Fund

A portion of the proceeds of the sale of *Grub* will go to the Grub Fund, which will be divided between b-healthy and the Small Planet Fund.

b-healthy | b-healthy.org

I founded b-healthy in 2001 to educate low-income youth about the connections between their personal health and the social and economic health of their communities. With a small team of dedicated staff and amazing volunteers, we provide low-income urban youth and youth organizations with resources to improve diet-related health in low-income communities; empower youth to understand the connections between food access, poverty, malnutrition, and institutional racism; and raise awareness about the need to improve individual and community health as a part of building broader movements for social justice.

BRYANT

Small Planet Institute and Small Planet Fund | smallplanetfund.org

My mother and I founded the Small Planet Institute to bring to light the emergence of living democracy. On every continent, people are discovering their power to act on their values and create communities that work for all. At the Institute we further this historic transition through books, articles, and other media as well as through the Small Planet Fund. Inspired by the courageous changemakers we met in writing *Hope's Edge,* we founded the Fund to support their much-needed work. The volunteer-run Fund channels resources raised through individual donations to grassroots organizations around the world addressing the root causes of hunger and poverty.

ANNA

Index

COMMUNITY FOOD AUDIT

Once you've created your community food audit, you can share it with friends, deliver it to your local café or community center, post it at your church. Spread the knowledge!
Visit eatgrub.org for more resources.

City/Neighborhood: _____

Farmers' market | sustainabletable.org and ams.usda.gov/farmersmarkets

_____

Location

_____   _____

Day(s)   *Hours*

CSA Farm | localharvest.org and csacenter.org

_____   _____

Name of Farm   *Name of Farmer(s)*

_____

Pick-up Location

_____   _____

Pick-up Day and Time   *Member Share ($) and Due Date*

Food Coop | cooperativegrocer.org

_____

Location

_____

Days/Hours of Operation

Grocery Stores with Local Foods | foodroutes.org

_____   _____

Name of Store   *Name of Store Manager or Food Buyer*

_____

Phone Number

Your Local Organic Meat and Dairy/Egg Provider | eatwellguide.org

(if you eat meat, and if your CSA doesn't offer meat or dairy)

_____   _____

Name of Farm   *Name of Farmer(s)*

_____

Phone Number

Community Garden | communitygarden.org

_____

Location

_____

Days/Hours of Operation

Elected Officials | congress.org

(Includes local, state, and federal elected officials and information on government agencies plus much more)

_____

_____

School Food Resources | farmtoschool.org and farmtocollege.org

(e.g., farm-to-school and farm-to-college efforts, school board members, healthy food in schools initiatives, wellness policy councils)

_____

_____

_____

Other Community Food Resources | foodsecurity.org

(e.g., local restaurants, community garden associations, buy-local campaigns, fair-trade certified providers, farmworker solidarity organizations, food policy councils)

_____

_____

_____